The Fat Flush Foods

Other Books in the Fat Flush Program

The Fat Flush Plan

The Fat Flush Cookbook

The Fat Flush Journal and Shopping Guide

The Complete Fat Flush Program

The Fat Flush Fitness Plan
(with Joanie Greggains)

The Fat Flush Foods

ANN LOUISE GITTLEMAN
M.S., C.N.S.

McGraw-Hill

New York / Chicago / San Francisco / Lisbon / London
Madrid / Mexico City / Milan / New Delhi / San Juan
Seoul / Singapore / Sydney / Toronto

The McGraw-Hill Companies

1 2 3 4 5 6 7 8 9 0 DOC/DOC 0 9 8 7 6 5 4

ISBN 0-07-144068-2

This book is for educational purposes. It is not intended as a substitute for medical advice. Please consult a qualified health care professional for individual health and medical advice. Neither McGraw-Hill nor the author shall have any responsibility for any adverse effects arising directly or indirectly as a result of the information provided in this book.

Throughout this book, trademarked names are used. Rather than put a trademark symbol after every occurrence of a trademarked name, we use names in an editorial fashion only and to the benefit of the trademark owner, with no intention of infringement of the trademark. Where such designations appear in this book, they have been printed with initial capitals.

McGraw-Hill books are available at special discounts to use as premiums and sales promotions, or for use in corporate training programs. For more information, please write to the Director of Special Sales, Professional Publishing, McGraw-Hill, Two Penn Plaza, New York, NY 10121-2298. Or contact your local bookstore.

This book is printed on recycled, acid-free paper containing a minimum of 50% recycled de-inked paper.

Library of Congress Cataloging-in-Publication Data

Gittleman, Ann Louise.
The fat flush foods : the world's best foods, seasonings, and supplements to flush the fat from every body / Ann Louise Gittleman.
p. cm.
Includes bibliographical references.
ISBN 0-07-144068-2 (pbk. : alk. paper)
1. Reducing diets. 2. Functional foods. I. Title.
RM222.2.G53725 2004
613.2'5—dc22

2004001376

Acknowledgments

My heartfelt thanks are extended to Fat Flushers throughout the world who have embraced my program so wholeheartedly and achieved such astounding weight loss and healing results. I especially want to acknowledge all my community leaders—both here and abroad—for their 24/7 never-ending support and virtual friendship. Linda L, Mary, Carol, LSue, Martha, Barbara, Kathy, Jackie, and Linda P.—you are simply the best.

Linda Leekley deserves a very special thank you for her creative assistance and continual devotion, dedication, and commitment, which always serve to remind me why I got into this business in the first place. Linda runs a full-time business but manages to oversee our FatFlush forum and coordinate Fat Flush outreach programs like our Fat Flush cruises. She is extraordinary.

Finally, thanks also to the entire editorial and production staff at McGraw Hill and the staff of First Lady, Inc. who have been with me since the debut of *The Fat Flush Plan*. What a wonderful ride it has been!

Contents

Introduction

It's true.

Combining the right kinds of foods in your diet does more for your figure than any weight loss "magic bullet" ever could. But, today we live in a constant state of information overload, and it can be overwhelming to try to decipher all the reports about which foods are slimming and which foods pack on the pounds. For example, to say that broccoli is good for you or that eggs contain cholesterol is hardly headline news. However, did you know that broccoli promotes weight loss by balancing blood-sugar levels and that over 200 scientific studies have proven that eating eggs does not boost cholesterol? These are just two of the fifty foods, spices, and supplements that I have chosen as twenty-first-century Fat Flushing "superfoods."

Nutritionally dense, a Fat Flushing superfood is a therapeutic bombshell that flushes fat from the body, detoxifies the body, and contributes to overall health and beauty. Because a healthy diet is the most important factor in losing weight and maintaining overall health, I've chosen the best of the best—the top 50 Fat Flushing foods, spices, and supplements that contribute to a fit, younger-looking body.

Based on the latest research, I've put together all you need to know about the premier foods known to burn fat, boost your metabolism, detoxify your body, and erase excess water weight, while controlling cholesterol and blood-sugar levels. In fact, I've categorized each of the 50 items so that you can know at a glance how they contribute to weight loss. Throughout this book, the following basic categories will guide you on your Fat Flush journey toward better health and fitness:

Blood-Sugar Stabilizer

Foods with this designation are known for steadying your blood sugar, which serves to curb your appetite and prevent the fatty deposits that are part of "insulin resistance."

Cholesterol Zapper

Foods that help rid the body of cholesterol or help balance the ratio between "good" and "bad" cholesterol levels are marked with this icon.

Detoxifier

To earn this designation, foods must be known for ridding the body of toxins, thereby creating a cleansed and invigorated liver, which is ready to function as a fat-burning machine.

Diuretic

Foods that help dewaterlog the tissues and eliminate excess water weight are marked with this icon.

Energizer

To carry this designation, a food must fight fatigue, ward off stress, and provide an energizing boost to the entire body.

Thermogenic

These are foods that raise body temperature, thereby helping it to burn fat efficiently rather than storing it as fuel.

I encourage you to become familiar with each of the 50 items detailed in this book. By peppering your grocery list with these Fat Flushing superfoods, you'll say goodbye to weight gain, bloating, and those stubborn fat deposits on your hips, thighs, and buttocks. However, this book is just one of the pieces of the Fat Flush puzzle. In addition, I invite you to explore the complete Fat Flush Plan, which details even further how to use these Fat Flushing foods to increase your metabolism, eliminate bloat, and speed up fat loss.

The Fat Flush Plan goes beyond the conventional answers by uncovering the root causes of why we gain weight. It is an exciting breakthrough program, already in use by millions of people who are discovering both short-term weight loss and long-term wellness. Yet, even with just this book as your companion, you can begin to eat your way to weight loss, beauty, and overall good health. By learning about these 50 Fat Flushing foods, spices, and supplements, you'll be informed and in control of gaining the fit, tight, healthy body you've always wanted.

CHAPTER

1 Fat Flushing Staples

The biggest room in the world is the room for improvement.

ANONYMOUS

My breakthrough eating program, the Fat Flush Plan, contains key elements—designated here as Fat Flushing Staples—which trigger both fat and weight loss safely and simply. Fat Flushers everywhere are discovering this new paradigm shift in weight loss and lasting weight control: The liver is the primary fat-burning organ in the body, and it must be cleansed and supported in order to achieve peak performance.

Your liver is strongly affected by a poor diet. In fact, a liver overloaded with pollutants and toxins is the number one weight-loss roadblock. Excess fat, sugar, alcohol, and caffeine—along with antidepressants and birth control pills—work to sabotage your weight-loss efforts by creating a tired and toxic liver that can't efficiently burn body fat. The Fat Flush Plan is designed to clean out the liver and help you drop a dress size or two in relatively short order.

This groundbreaking diet doesn't stop at flushing fat. Fat Flushers have also found that it improves circulation, increases energy, stabilizes mood swings, induces sound sleep, improves skin texture, makes nails stronger, and helps to lessen depression and anxiety. They also report lower cholesterol (as much as 30 points) and balanced triglyceride levels. In addition, the added bonus of internal cleansing provides unexpected mental and emotional benefits. A clean body translates into clearer thinking and mental alertness.

The six Fat Flushing Staples detailed in this chapter are crucial to the success enjoyed by many Fat Flushers around the globe. From the initial 2-week detoxification phase to the second phase of ongoing weight loss to the third phase of lifestyle eating, the Fat Flush Plan depends on each of the following six superfoods to perform its individual magic. And, by working together, these Fat Flushing Staples transform your shape by rejuvenating the liver and accelerating fat loss from your body's favorite fat storage areas—your hips, thighs, and buttocks.

APPLE CIDER VINEGAR

Fat Flush Factors

Thermogenic

Detoxifier

Cholesterol Zapper

Energizer

An excellent fat burner, apple cider vinegar (ACV) helps whittle away excess weight and revs up the metabolism. In fact, a recent Arizona State University study found that participants who consumed as little as 1½ tablespoons of apple cider vinegar ate 200 fewer calories at the following meal.[1] That's amazing, considering that apple cider vinegar, or ACV, is nothing more than freshly pressed apple juice that has fermented at room temperature for a few weeks.

The main ingredient in apple cider vinegar, acetic acid, is a powerful nutrient that has been proven to stimulate the metabolism. ACV also contains dozens of other nutrients that work to eliminate fat by creating the ideal chemical balance in the body. Researchers at the University of Sydney found that consuming vinegar with meals can lower blood sugar by as much as 30 percent.[2] The acidity in ACV helps slow stomach emptying, which means that food takes longer to reach your small intestine and bloodstream. As a result, carbohydrates are digested more slowly, thereby lowering blood-sugar levels and keeping the appetite in check.

Apple cider vinegar contains potassium, which helps transfer nutrients to your cells and give toxic waste substances the boot. The beta-carotene found in ACV also helps cleanse the body by getting rid of free radicals, those unstable molecules that can damage fat, protein, and even our DNA. In a spoonful of cider vinegar, you'll also find pectin, a fiber that "scrapes" the cholesterol off blood vessel walls. ACV is also full of enzymes and amino acids that assist in the development of healthy protein in the body. Studies in Japan have demonstrated that ACV reduces cholesterol and slows down the aging process by destroying free radicals in the body.[3]

Could there possibly be more? You bet. Apple cider vinegar helps cleanse and tone the digestive tract, increases circulation, soothes achy joints and sore muscles, and gives skin a healthy sheen. Pick up a bottle of apple cider vinegar today, and you'll be on your way to a lighter and lovelier you!

Recommended Usage: Up to 2 teaspoons per day, mixed with water, in recipes or as a salad dressing.

Just the Facts

- In 400 B.C., Hippocrates, the father of medicine, recognized the powerful cleansing, healing, and germ-fighting qualities of apple cider vinegar.
- Apple cider vinegar makes a terrific pH-balancing bath and adds shine when used as a hair rinse.

Boost the Benefits

- When shopping for cider vinegar, look for brands that are certified organic, unfiltered, and unpasteurized. Read the label carefully because some companies sell apple cider "flavored" vinegar.
- Apple cider vinegar requires no additives or preservatives. And there's no need to worry about bacteria such as E. coli affecting ACV (the way it might affect apple juice) since E. coli can't survive in vinegar's acidic environment.
- Apple cider vinegar should be a rich brownish color with visible sediment. The cobweblike strands floating in a bottle of natural ACV are edible protein substances that are referred to as the "mother." Having a "mother" in your bottle of cider vinegar is a *good* thing because it indicates that the vinegar is all natural.
- Organic ACV has a pleasant, but pungent, odor and taste, sometimes causing you to pucker up.
- Store your apple cider vinegar in a dark cupboard to protect the vital nutrients.

Fat Flush in Action

- Make a thirst-quenching drink by mixing a teaspoon of apple cider vinegar with a tall glass of water.
- Before cooking, soak fish in apple cider vinegar and water for a tender, sweeter taste.
- To create a fluffy meringue, beat 3 egg whites with a teaspoon of ACV.
- To tenderize meat, marinate it overnight in apple cider vinegar and your favorite herbs and spices.

It's Been Said . . .

Apple cider vinegar and flax oil make a terrific salad dressing. I use it every day and have lost 25 pounds in three months.

ELAINE T., TEXAS

CRANBERRIES

Fat Flush Factors

Diuretic

Detoxifier

Cholesterol Zapper

Native to North America, the cranberry can still be found growing wild in the cool, sandy bogs of Massachusetts and New Jersey. It was Dutch and German settlers who named this bright red berry, calling it "crane" berry after the birdlike shape of its blossoms.

Cranberries—and pure, unsweetened cranberry juice—enjoy superstar status as a prime component of the Fat Flush Plan. Cranberries contain significant amounts of both *flavonoids* and *polyphenolic compounds,* shown to prevent the oxidation of LDL cholesterol. LDL cholesterol is the "bad" type of cholesterol, which becomes dangerous to the body only after it has been oxidized. Ongoing research continues to suggest that cranberries offer a natural defense against atherosclerosis and heart disease. At the Technical University of Denmark, researchers compared the health benefits of cranberry and blueberry juice. The results? Cranberries won, hands down. In fact, while cranberry juice proved to be a powerful antioxidant, blueberry juice served up no more nutritional benefit than sugar water.[4]

Only a few years ago, some doctors discounted cranberry juice as a natural prevention for bladder infections. Now, thanks to research conducted by the Harvard Medical School and Rutgers University, physicians know that cranberries help prevent the bacteria, E. coli, from sticking to the lining of the bladder.[5] The news gets even better. It turns out that cranberries have a similar effect in the mouth, preventing bacteria from gathering on the surface of your teeth where it can cause gingivitis and periodontal disease.[6] The antibacterial power of cranberries also shows up in the stomach, providing much needed protection against the ulcer-causing bacterium H. pylori.[7]

All these health improvements make cranberries worth every penny. However, Fat Flushers know that cranberries offer another very important side effect. Pure cranberry juice is absorbed immediately into the system, where it helps keep your liver's detoxification pathways open, provides antioxidants called phenols, along with vitamin-C–related bioflavonoids to strengthen your connective tissue, and, based on my observations over the past 15 years, acts as a digestive aid for any stubborn fat deposits remaining in your lymphatic system. This could well be the reason why people on the Fat Flush Plan see their cellulite disappear.

So expand your consumption of cranberries *beyond* the Thanksgiving holiday, and you'll gain an abundance of health—and beauty—benefits all year long.

Recommended Usage: One cup of 100 percent pure, unsweetened cranberry juice per day.

Just the Facts

- In colonial times, cranberries did triple duty as a medicine, a colorful natural dye, and as a symbol of peace.
- Cranberries are one of only three original American fruits still being produced today, with nearly 600 million pounds harvested every October. If you strung together all the cranberries produced in North America last year, they would stretch from Boston to Los Angeles more than 565 times!
- Cranberries are considered a "functional" food, meaning they provide natural health benefits far beyond basic nutrition.
- Based on serving size, pure, unsweetened cranberry juice has the highest antioxidant level of any cranberry product.
- Cranberry juice helps prevent a vitamin B^{12} deficiency by increasing the body's absorption of this important nutrient.

Boost the Benefits

- When shopping for cranberries, look for fruit that is shiny and plump and that has a bright color. A good quality, ripe cranberry will bounce.
- You may store cranberries in the refrigerator in their original, unopened plastic bags for 1 or 2 months. They may be kept frozen for 8 to 9 months. Once cooked, they will stay fresh for up to a month in a covered container in the refrigerator.
- Because overcooking gives them a bitter taste, cranberries should be cooked only until they "pop."

THINK TWICE!

When buying cranberry juice, remember to read labels carefully. The wording on the label provides strong clues to the content. For exam-

ple, a cranberry "drink" or "cocktail" usually contains ample amounts of sugar water or corn syrup, with a little real juice thrown in for good measure. Bottles marked "no sugar added" are often sweetened with apple or grape juice. For maximum Fat Flushing benefit, look for 100 percent pure, unsweetened cranberry juice.

It's Been Said . . .

For my entire life, my thighs bulged out at the sides. . . I was the ultimate pear shape. Now my sides are straight and firm. I've been dieting off and on ever since I was in junior high and this has NEVER happened before. I believe it's the daily cranberry juice mixed with water that helps the most. I could tell a real difference even in the first week or two of drinking it and now if I get little or no cran-water when I travel, I really miss that cleaned-out leaner feeling I get while I'm drinking it.

KATHY J., NEW YORK

FLAXSEED OIL

Fat Flush Factors

Cholesterol Zapper

Energizer

Blood-Sugar Stabilizer

Detoxifier

For Fat Flushers, flaxseed oil is a key element, capable of setting off a domino effect of weight loss and health benefits. It contains omega-3 *(essential fatty acids),* which, along with CLA and GLA, are the missing links to health, beauty and weight loss. As their name implies, essential fatty acids are vital for human health, but, because they cannot be made by the body, they must be obtained from foods. If your waistline is expanding, it could be because of a deficiency in the right kind of fat!

An omega-3 deficiency promotes weight gain in several ways. First, the appetite center in your brain may not be getting the message that you are full, so you eat more than you need. Second, your metabolism slows down, causing you to take in more calories than you burn off. By consuming flaxseed oil, you'll feel full for up for 3 or 4 hours so you won't be tempted to overeat between meals. Also, the omega-3's in the flaxseed oil are known to boost seratonin levels in the brain. As a result, you won't feel depressed, and you won't feel the need to eat to release anxiety and stress. And flaxseed oil revs up your metabolism, stimulates bile production, and attracts oil-soluble toxins that have been lodged in fatty tissues in the body, eliminating them from your system.

Beyond being a dieter's dream, flaxseed oil plays a critical role in healthy brain function, proper thyroid and adrenal activity, and balanced hormones. It strengthens the immune system, helps maintain healthy blood and nerves, and breaks down cholesterol. The omega-3's in flaxseed oil are also needed to produce flexible cell membranes, which allow for efficient use of insulin and stabilization of blood sugar. In the colon, omega-3 fats help protect colon cells from cancer-causing toxins and free radicals, thus reducing the risk of colon cancer. And, on the beauty front, flaxseed oil promotes glowing skin, shiny hair, and strong nails.

You can see why I consider flaxseed oil so vital to everyone's health and wellness. Is it any wonder that this precious oil has been nicknamed "liquid gold"? Do yourself a favor—get over your fear of fat and add flaxseed oil to your daily diet. You'll pare off the pounds and develop that Fat Flushing "glow"!

Recommended Usage: Two tablespoons of flaxseed oil per day.

Just the Facts

- Flax plants grow well in most climates, except for areas with searing hot or bitterly cold weather.
- After settling in North America, most colonists made planting flax a top priority.
- For centuries, freshly pressed flaxseed oil was sold by street vendors in northern Europe.
- Dry skin is the first—and most common—sign that you are deficient in omega-3 fatty acids.

Boost the Benefits

- Flaxseed oil is highly perishable and should be purchased in opaque bottles that have been kept refrigerated.
- Because heat destroys the sensitive fatty acids in flaxseed oil, you cannot cook or bake with it. Avoid direct exposure to heat.
- Fresh flaxseed oil has a sweet, nutty flavor. It can vary from brand to brand, so be sure to try several to find the one that suits you best.
- By blending flaxseed oil with other foods, rather than taking it alone by the spoonful, you allow it to emulsify, which ensures better absorption of the essential fatty acids.

Be a Fat Flush Cook

- Add a tablespoon of flaxseed oil to your breakfast smoothie. Your appetite will be satisfied for hours!
- Mix yogurt and flaxseed oil for a healthy alternative to mayonnaise.
- For people on the Fat Flush Plan, butter is a Phase 3 treat. To give your Phase 3 butter a bigger nutritional bite, try making a flavorful flax spread. Melt a stick of butter and remove it from the heat. Add 4 ounces of flaxseed oil and stir until blended. Pour the mixture into a container, cover it, and store in the refrigerator until it solidifies.
- For a great Phase 3 snack, mix 1 tablespoon of flaxseed oil into a cup of yogurt, and add your favorite fruit.

- Drizzle flaxseed oil over steamed veggies, and then sprinkle with your favorite herbs. In fact, flaxseed oil may be added to any food after the food has been heated.

THINK TWICE!

If flaxseed oil tastes harsh, is intensely bitter, or feels scratchy to your throat, it is old and should be discarded.

FLAXSEEDS

Fat Flush Factors

Cholesterol Zapper

Blood-Sugar Stabilizer

Detoxifier

One of people's earliest food supplies, flaxseeds definitely live up to their Latin name, *Linum usitatissium,* which means "most useful." These tiny brown seeds may not look like much, but they are held dear by Fat Flushers all over the globe for their omega-3 content and exceptional health benefits.

Slightly larger than sesame seeds, flaxseeds taste sweet and somewhat nutty. They contain 40 percent oil and are the number one source of ALA, alpha linolenic acid, an essential fatty acid required for efficient metabolism. Flaxseeds are also a superior source of lignans, plant estrogens known for their ability to fight cancer, keep viruses at bay, and balance hormone levels. Ounce for ounce, flaxseeds contain 800 times as many lignans as any other plant.

Lignan-rich flaxseeds have also been shown to reduce insulin resistance, which, in turn, has a positive impact on estrogen levels and breast cancer risk. And since insulin resistance is an early warning sign for type-2 diabetes, flaxseeds may also provide protection against this disease, which is currently a U.S. epidemic.[8]

When flaxseeds come in contact with liquid, they become soft and jellylike, making them highly useful as an intestinal cleanser and bowel regulator. The *soluble* fiber in flaxseeds helps reduce the amount of carbohydrates absorbed by our bodies. In addition, it stabilizes blood-sugar levels, minimizes cholesterol absorption, and lowers cholesterol levels. And, the 5 grams of *insoluble* fiber per tablespoon help ease elimination by absorbing water in the intestinal tract. In addition, flaxseeds contain *prussic acid,* which improves digestion. Be sure to take advantage of the healthy "scrubbing action" this Fat Flushing superfood has to offer!

Recommended Usage: Two tablespoons of ground flaxseeds per day.

Just the Facts

- Currently, Canada is the major producer of flaxseeds.
- The only difference between brown and golden flaxseeds is their color.
- As a source of plant sterols, flaxseeds boost immune function.

Boost the Benefits

- You may purchase flaxseeds either whole or already ground. While ground flaxseeds may be more convenient, whole flaxseeds have a longer shelf life.
- Whole flaxseeds can be found in prepackaged containers as well as in bulk bins. If you purchase them from a bulk bin, make sure the bin is covered and has no signs of moisture.
- Don't consume whole flaxseeds, or you'll miss out on important nutrients. The lignans are found in the fibrous shell hull of the flaxseeds and are only released when the seeds are ground.
- If you purchase whole flaxseeds, store them in an airtight container in a dark, dry, cool place where they should maintain their freshness for several months.
- Packages of preground flaxseeds should be vacuum-packed and/or refrigerated because, at room temperature, ground flaxseed spoils within just a few days.
- If you grind flaxseeds at home, keep them in a tightly sealed container in the refrigerator or freezer to prevent them from becoming rancid.
- To extend the freshness, you may freeze both whole and ground flaxseeds for up to 1 year.
- To grind whole flaxseeds, try a coffee or seed grinder. You'll have beautifully ground flaxseeds at the push of a button!

Be a Fat Flush Cook

- Sprinkle ground flaxseeds onto a variety of foods, from yogurt to salads to steamed veggies to a bowl of soup.
- Add flaxseeds to your homemade muffin, cookie, or bread recipes. But remember not to set your oven temperature higher than 350 degrees.
- To pump up the nutritional volume of your breakfast shake, add ground flaxseeds.
- To give sliced fruit a nuttier flavor, sprinkle some ground flaxseeds on top of it.

THINK TWICE!

Flaxseeds contain cyanogenic glycosides, naturally occurring plant compounds, which, in large amounts, can suppress the thyroid's ability to take up sufficient iodine. To deactivate the glycosides, toast your whole flaxseeds for 15 minutes in a 250 degree oven prior to grinding them.

It's Been Said . . .

Every morning and every evening, I mix ground flaxseeds, unsweetened cranberry juice, and water to make a Fat Flushing Long Life Cocktail. I love the nutty flavor of the flaxseeds, and it's great knowing that something so simple is working to improve my health!

DEBBIE R., IDAHO

LEMONS

Fat Flush Factors

Cholesterol Zapper

Detoxifier

Diuretic

Thermogenic

Originally developed as a cross between a lime and a citron, lemons first appeared in China over 2000 years ago. Christopher Columbus brought lemons to the Americas, and they have been grown in Florida ever since! Many people think of lemons only in terms of lemonade, but, nutritionally, this little yellow fruit can do much more than quench your thirst on a hot summer day.

Lemons are high in vitamin C, supplying four times more than oranges. As the primary water-soluble antioxidant in the body, vitamin C travels through your system, preventing cellular damage and cholesterol buildup by zapping any free radicals it meets. Recently, researchers discovered a substance in lemons called *limonene*. This essential oil has been shown to shrink cancerous tumors, detoxify carcinogens in the body, and stimulate the healthy flow of lymph fluids.

Lemons assist in the digestive process by producing necessary enzymes, invigorating the gall bladder and liver, and promoting the absorption of protein and minerals from foods. Lemon juice also helps liquefy fat so that it can be flushed out of your system faster. And, as if that weren't enough, drinking lemon juice in hot water acts as a mild diuretic, ridding the body of retained water and toxins. It may also help to reduce cellulite by cleansing the lymphatic system and stimulating blood flow to the skin.

To top it off, lemons also provide small amounts of vitamin B^6, potassium, calcium, magnesium, and folate. So, run, don't walk, to pick up this Fat Flushing superfood today!

Recommended Usage: The juice of at least one lemon every day.

Just the Facts

- Unlike oranges, lemons continue to ripen even after they are picked.

- Consuming lemons with sugar negates many of the health benefits of the fruit. The sugar lowers immunity, interferes with digestion, and leeches vitamins and minerals from the body.
- Aromatherapists believe that the smell of a lemon is beneficial because it helps reduce feelings of stress and boosts the immune system.
- Much of the taste and aroma of a lemon comes from the "zest"—oils that are abundant in the fruit's peel.

Boost the Benefits

- To find a good-quality lemon, remember that the thinner the skin, the more flesh the lemon will have—and the juicier it will be. Look for firm, fine-textured lemons that are heavy for their size.
- Pick lemons with a bright yellow color, because the ones with a green tinge are not fully ripe and will be more acidic.
- Lemons are *overripe* if they are wrinkled, reddish in color, or have soft or hard patches.
- If you plan to use the skin or zest of the lemon, choose fruit that is certified organic to avoid exposure to pesticides and wax.
- As long as they are protected from sunlight, lemons will stay fresh at room temperature for about 1 week.
- To keep lemons longer, store them in the refrigerator crisper where they will keep for about 4 weeks.
- Use a lemon as quickly as possible after cutting it.
- Since lemons produce more juice when they are warm, bring them to room temperature before juicing them by placing them in a bowl of warm water for several minutes. Rolling a lemon under the palm of your hand on a hard surface also produces more juice.
- Lemon juice can be frozen. Place freshly squeezed lemon juice in ice-cube trays until frozen. Then store the lemon cubes in plastic bags in the freezer until they are needed.

Be a Fat Flush Cook

- Combine lemon juice with olive or flaxseed oil, freshly crushed garlic, and cayenne to make a zesty salad dressing.
- Because acids help proteins coagulate, your poached eggs will keep their shape if you add a few drops of lemon juice to the cooking water.
- Squirt lemon juice on cut fruits or white vegetables to help them keep their color.
- When preparing fish, place thin lemon slices underneath and around the fish. As the fish bakes or broils, the lemon slices will soften and may be eaten along with the fish.

- That glass of water will have more zip and look prettier if you add a slice of lemon to it.

THINK TWICE!

When preparing recipes that include lemons or lemon juice, use nonreactive cookware, such as stainless steel, enamel, or plastic. Exposing lemon to uncoated iron, copper, or aluminum cookware can discolor the food and leave a metallic taste.

It's Been Said . . .

First, I learned to "lemonize" my foods. Now, I serve lemon wedges with all my meals. Squeezing lemon juice on my foods serves as a great salt substitute and really helps to cut the fat. Give it a try!

ELLEN H., NORTH CAROLINA

I come from a long line of cellulite-prone women, so you can imagine how happy I was to find a way to eliminate it! I figured that if the cellulite went away, any additional weight loss would be a bonus. The majority of my cellulite disappeared in the first two weeks of following the Fat Flush Plan, including the hot lemon water every morning. Even though I didn't get on a scale, I could see my thighs shrinking. I'm one happy woman!

CHARLI S., WASHINGTON

WATER

Fat Flush Factors

Detoxifier

Diuretic

Thermogenic

Did you know that the average person loses 10 cups of water each day just by breathing, perspiring, and using the bathroom? Yet, a recent survey conducted by the International Bottled Water Association found that most Americans drink no more than 5 cups of water a day. While additional water is absorbed from the foods we eat, the math still doesn't add up, especially when many people counteract their intake of water by consuming caffeine-filled teas, coffees, or sodas, which inhibit the reabsorption of water. It's no wonder that a Cornell University survey showed that 75 percent of Americans are chronically dehydrated![9]

Even mild dehydration, such as a 2 percent drop in body water, can produce problems, including memory deficits, an inability to focus, and daytime fatigue. Some subtle signs of dehydration include dry lips, dark colored urine, muscle or joint soreness, headaches, crankiness, fatigue, and constipation. Ironically, if you don't drink enough water, your body senses trouble and begins to hang on to every bit of water it can. If you fail to hydrate your body, it stores water between cells and you end up carrying excess water weight.

To make matters worse, if you are dehydrated, your body stores more fat. Why? Without water, your kidneys are forced to call on the liver to help perform their functions. This keeps the liver from being able to burn as much fat as it normally would, so the fat gets deposited—often around the belly. In addition to reducing fat deposits and ridding the body of toxins, consuming generous amounts of water is an effective way to reduce cravings. Because water is a natural appetite suppressant and helps you feel full, you may not feel hungry if you drink it regularly throughout the day.

Still not convinced? Keep in mind that water is a powerful tool for a clear, beautiful complexion. Your body prioritizes where the water goes, and since vital organs take precedence, your skin is last on the list. If you fail to drink enough water, your skin will suffer more than any other part of your body. Being well hydrated also helps reduce constipation and, because water allows for efficient elimination, has even been shown to decrease the risk of colon cancer by 45 percent. Furthermore, a 2002 study concluded that a daily intake of at least five glasses of water cut the risk of heart disease in half![10] So, "Bottoms up" to all my Fat Flushing friends.

Recommended Usage: Eight 8-ounce glasses of water per day, plus one 8-ounce glass for each hour of light activity.

Just the Facts

- The human body is nearly 70 percent water. This amount can be seriously affected by stress, alcohol, and caffeine.
- While people can live without food for about a month, they can't last a week without water.
- If you wait until you are thirsty to drink some water, you will already be dehydrated! By the time you feel thirsty you have already lost over 1 percent of your total body water.

Boost the Benefits

- Keep a bottle of water with you in the car so that you can grab a few sips while you're on the run.
- Don't drink ice water with meals as it dilutes digestive enzymes. To enhance digestion, enjoy a cup of hot water with lemon immediately after your meal.
- Caffeinated coffees, teas, and sodas are no substitute for water, since caffeine functions as a diuretic, causing you to lose water through frequent urination.
- Because your body loses water while you sleep, it's a great idea to start and end your day with a glass of water.
- Keep drinking while you exercise! By replacing the fluid you lose as sweat, water keeps your energy level stable during exercise. Since water plays an important role in the transport of nutrients and chemical reactions in the body, staying hydrated boosts the metabolism, increasing the number of calories burnt during daily activities. So, have a bottle of water handy and take frequent water breaks.

Be a Fat Flush Cook

- Adding ice cubes to your morning smoothie creates a thick drink with the power to hydrate.

- Make water-filled foods a regular part of your diet. These include broth-based soups, lettuce, broccoli, and citrus fruits.
- Wean yourself off of regular juice by diluting it with water, adding less and less juice as time goes on.
- To entice yourself (and your family members) to drink more water, try some of the following tips:
    - Add a splash of lemon juice to your water for a tangy flavor.
    - Make juice cubes by filling an ice-cube tray with lemon or cranberry juice. Pop a cube or two into a tall glass of water for a refreshing, festive drink.
    - Drop a couple of frozen strawberries into your water.

CHAPTER

2 Fat Flushing Proteins

Every day, do something that will inch you closer to a better tomorrow.

DOUG FIREBAUGH

Composed of amino acids, protein is vital as a "building block" for every human cell. It also maintains proper fluid balance, supports hormone and enzyme development, enhances the immune system, and, of course, provides energy to every part of the body. Since our bodies can't store protein, it must be supplied on a daily basis from the foods we eat. And, while proteins are found in all types of foods, only meat, eggs, and other foods from animal sources contain *complete* proteins, which provide all eight essential amino acids.

Unfortunately, many people have a media-driven fear of fat, which extends to a fear of eating certain proteins. You needn't worry about any of my five Fat Flushing protein selections presented in this chapter hindering your health or weight loss. For example, beef is included as a Fat Flushing superfood because it is the highest dietary source of l-carnitine, an incredibly effective fat-burning nutrient. And eggs have been found innocent of raising cholesterol levels. In fact, the *Journal of the American Medical Association* published results of an 8-year study that tracked nearly 40,000 men and 80,000 women and showed there was no link between egg consumption and the risk of coronary heart disease.

The protein-rich Fat Flushing superfoods found in this chapter are important weight loss tools. Protein helps you feel full faster and requires more energy to digest than other foods, thereby using up more calories and contributing to weight loss. In fact, by building muscle mass, protein has been shown to raise your metabolism by nearly 30 percent,[1] which gears up your calorie-burning thyroid gland. By slowing down the absorption of glucose into the bloodstream, protein stabilizes your blood-sugar level. And, as you flush more and more fat, protein-rich foods will help preserve your all-important lean muscle tissue.

BEEF

Fat Flush Factors

Energizer

Thermogenic

For years, the media gave beef a bad rap, causing many people to shy away from buying even the leanest cuts of beef. Much to my delight, the current popularity of high-protein diets has boosted sales of beef across America, yet we still consume 25 percent less beef than we did in the mid-1970s. When was the last time you enjoyed some beef? I'm not talking about a fast-food hamburger, but rather a lean, tasty piece of steak, fillet, or roast. This nutrient-rich food promotes a strong immune system, provides energy to every cell, and helps build those all-important fat-burning muscles.

Beef is hearty and deeply flavored and ranks high as a source for protein, vitamin B^{12}, zinc, and the potent Fat Flushing fat-burner, l-carnitine. A 3-ounce serving of beef supplies as much iron as 3 cups of raw spinach and as much zinc as 30 ounces of tuna. Beef also ranks high in iron, phosphorus, selenium and the B-complex vitamins. In addition, about half the fat in beef is healthy monounsaturated fat, which does not raise cholesterol levels.

Beef's vitamin B^{12} content helps the body convert the potentially dangerous chemical *homocysteine* into harmless molecules, decreasing the risk of heart attack, stroke, and even osteoporosis. Organic beef is also a very good source of the trace mineral selenium, which helps reduce the risk of colon cancer and supports antioxidant activity in the liver and throughout the body. In addition, the zinc in lean beef helps prevent blood vessel damage that can lead to atherosclerosis and is also needed for proper functioning of the immune system.

Most of the beef available today is raised on grass and fattened on feed lots with feed consisting of corn and molasses, plus a hefty dose of antibiotics and other additives. For meat that is free of antibiotics, added hormones, and pesticides, consider buying organically certified beef. Another option is to look for grass-fed beef, which is rich in essential fatty acids, vitamin E, and beta-carotene. (You'll find an extensive list of grass-fed beef providers in my book, the *Fat Flush Plan.*) Grass-fed beef contains significant amounts of two "good" fats, monounsaturated oils and stearic acid, but no artificial trans-fatty acids. Grass-fed beef is also the richest known natural source of CLA and is lower in total fat and calories than conventional beef.

Recommended Usage: Up to four 4-ounce servings per week.

Just the Facts

- At least a dozen cuts of beef are leaner than a skinless chicken thigh, including a sirloin steak, round steak, flank steak, tenderloin, tritip roast, and rump roast.
- Meat labeled "prime" is tender and juicy, but is generally higher in fat than other grades of meat.
- A 4-ounce serving of lean beef provides over 60 percent of the daily requirement for protein.
- A recent study published in the *Journal of Animal Science* concluded that a serving of grass-fed beef has less cholesterol than the same amount of chicken breast.[2]

Boost the Benefits

- At the grocery store, make raw beef the last item added to your grocery cart. Put the meat packages in plastic bags to keep juices from dripping onto other foods.
- Always check the sell-by date on the label and choose the beef with the latest date.
- Look for beef with a bright cherry-red color. Steaks and roasts should feel firm, not mushy.
- Go for the beef with the least amount of fat. Any fat on the meat should be white in color, not yellow, since meat with yellow fat is usually less tender.
- For the freshest and leanest ground beef, select a round or sirloin steak and ask the butcher to grind it for you.
- Refrigerate or freeze fresh beef immediately. Never leave beef sitting out at room temperature. Whole cuts of beef may be refrigerated in the coldest part of the refrigerator for 3 to 5 days, while refrigerated ground beef should be used within 1 or 2 days.
- To freeze beef, wrap it tightly in freezer paper. Ground beef should keep for about 3 months, and whole cuts are good for 6 months.
- Thaw frozen beef in the refrigerator or in cold water—never at room temperature. Likewise, you should marinate beef in the refrigerator, not on the counter.

- Food safety experts recommend using a thermometer to check for the "doneness" of cooked beef. The internal temperature of the meat should be at least 160 degrees.

THINK TWICE!

- Always *wash your hands thoroughly with hot soapy water after you handle raw beef.*
- *After handling raw beef, sanitize counters, cutting boards, and other surfaces with a solution of 1 teaspoon chlorine bleach per quart of water.*
- *Discard beef that is beginning to smell or if you feel it may be getting too old. Freezing it will* not *kill harmful bacteria.*

Be a Fat Flush Cook

- If you use grass-fed beef with its extremely low fat content, brush it with a bit of virgin olive oil to prevent drying and sticking. And keep in mind that it requires about 30 percent less cooking time than conventional beef.
- Sauté thin slices of steak or some lean ground beef in a bit of broth with onions and garlic. Add some no-salt tomato sauce or fresh tomatoes and serve over spaghetti squash.
- Skewer cubes of beef with your favorite Fat Flushing vegetables. Brush with a little olive oil and grill.
- Thinly sliced cooked tenderloin makes for a wonderful sandwich. Top it with onion slices and a crisp leaf of Romaine lettuce.
- Try a spice rub made up of your favorite Fat Flushing herbs and spices. Just rub the mixture on the meat prior to cooking.
- To allow the juices to redistribute, let cooked beef sit, covered and in a warm place, for about 10 minutes after removing it from the heat.
- To preserve juiciness, avoid piercing meat with a fork. Instead, always use tongs to turn your beef.

EGGS

Fat Flush Factors

Energizer

Blood-Sugar Stabilizer

An egg is one of nature's most nutritious creations. Except for vitamin C, eggs provide a perfect balance of every important vitamin and mineral. In addition, eggs are protein-rich, inexpensive, and delicious. For many years, eggs got a bad rap because of their cholesterol content. Yet people who eat only egg whites and skip the yolks are really missing out. While it's true that the egg yolk contains all the fat, it also provides nearly half the protein and most of the vitamins. And, while eggs are high in cholesterol, researchers have determined—in over 200 studies spanning the past 25 years—that it is not cholesterol, but rather the amount of *saturated fat* in foods that affects cholesterol levels.

Recently, the "classic" egg has been improved upon, and we can now purchase eggs that have a higher content of omega-3, a polyunsaturated fatty acid known to reduce blood triglyceride levels and the risk of heart disease. Omega-3–enriched eggs come from hens that are fed a special diet of ground flaxseed, which is higher in omega-3 fatty acids and lower in saturated fatty acids than other grains.

In addition, eggs are a great source of choline, a key nutrient required for brain function and nervous system health. Choline also affects cardiovascular health since it helps convert harmful homocysteine molecules into a benign substance. Eggs also contain a hefty supply of biotin, a B vitamin involved in producing energy by metabolizing both sugar and fat. Enjoy eggs for breakfast and you'll be energizing your body and pumping up your muscle tone.

When it comes to convenience and ease of preparation, eggs really are the best protein money can buy, and, because they provide more nutrients than calories, they earn the title, "nutrient dense." Omega-3–enriched eggs, such as Eggland's Best, are available in most grocery stores across America. Why not add a dozen to your grocery list today?

Recommended Usage: Up to two eggs per day, preferably omega-3–enriched eggs.

Just the Facts

- There is no nutritional difference between white and brown eggs. However, if you make hard-boiled eggs frequently, select brown eggs. They have a thicker shell and won't crack as easily.
- Two omega-3–enriched eggs provide about half of the recommended daily intake of omega-3 fatty acids.
- Eggs contain the highest quality of food protein known, second only to mother's milk.
- If you happen to drop an egg, cover it with salt and wait about ten minutes. Clean up will be a breeze!

Boost the Benefits

- When shopping for eggs, open the carton and make sure the eggs are clean and the shells aren't cracked.
- It's fine to buy organic, or free-range, eggs, but look for the words "omega-3–enriched" on the carton. Not all organic eggs are high in omega-3 fatty acids.
- Keep eggs refrigerated at all times, and they will maintain their freshness for several weeks. In fact, properly stored, eggs rarely spoil. If you keep them long enough, they are likely to simply dry up. However, at room temperature, eggs age more in one day than they do in one week in the refrigerator.
- Keep eggs in their original carton so that they do not lose moisture or pick up odors and flavors from other foods. Do not store them in the refrigerator door since repeated opening of the door exposes them to too much heat.
- Do not use an egg if it is cracked or leaking.
- After making hard-boiled eggs, store them in their shells, in the original carton. Use them within 1 week. And, if you notice a "gassy" odor in your refrigerator, remember that it is harmless and will disappear in a few hours. The smell comes from the hydrogen sulfide formed when eggs are hard-boiled.
- To freeze raw eggs, beat them until blended, pour them into a freezer container, seal it tightly, and freeze. But don't freeze hard-boiled eggs because freezing will make them tough and watery.

THINK TWICE!

- *To eliminate concern about eggshells carrying bacteria, clean your eggs with a Clorox wash. (See page 136.)*
- Always *wash your hands with warm, soapy water after contact with raw eggs.*

Be a Fat Flush Cook

- Hard-boiled eggs make a great snack and are easy to pack for on-the-go lunches.
- To cook eggs without added fat, try poaching them or use a non-stick pan with a bit of broth.
- For a healthy egg salad, chop some hard-boiled eggs and mix them with fresh lemon juice, flaxseed oil, minced onion, and dill.
- Serve a poached egg on a bed of steamed spinach for a vitamin-packed meal.
- Top scrambled eggs with homemade or organic salsa for a zesty breakfast.

Fat Flush Fun

Take your eggs and place them in a bowl of water. A fresh egg will sink to the bottom and lie on its side, while an older egg will stand up on one end. If the egg is really old, it may even float.

It's Been Said . . .

"I've been eating two omega-3 enriched eggs per day for over 6 months. Recently, I had my cholesterol checked, and it was back to normal—for the first time in years. Both my LDL and HDL levels were great and my triglycerides were 91. Hurray!"

BARBARA A., KENTUCKY

LAMB

Fat Flush Factors

Energizer

Blood-Sugar Stabilizer

Sheep have been a source of food and wool for thousands of years and are currently the most abundant livestock in the world. Lamb is a dietary staple throughout the world, including the Middle East, New Zealand, and Australia. Yet, throughout the United States, lamb has always taken a backseat to beef, pork, and veal. Statistics show that the average American consumes just over half a pound of lamb per year.

If you breeze by the lamb section every time you shop for groceries, you may want to reconsider. Lamb is lean and meaty and, unlike most red meats, is not "marbled" with saturated fat. Approximately 36 percent of the fat in lamb is saturated. The rest is mono- or polyunsaturated—the "good" type of dietary fat.

As a nutritionally complete protein, lamb provides all eight amino acids in the proper ratio. Lamb boosts your immune system and encourages growth and healing by providing an ample amount of zinc. Zinc also helps maintains a steady blood-sugar level and metabolic rate. Lamb energizes the body by supplying *heme iron*, a form of iron that is easily absorbed. On top of offering copper, manganese, selenium, and riboflavin, lamb is a good source of vitamin B^{12}, which helps the body metabolize nutrients and prevents anemia by building red blood cells.

Recommended Usage: One or two servings of lamb per week.

Just the Facts

- Lamb is the meat from young sheep that are less than 1 year old.
- If you buy graded lamb, remember that prime and choice cuts are the most tender and tasty, but also have the higher fat content.
- Free range lambs have a much finer texture and taste than those fed with grain.

Boost the Benefits

- When purchasing lamb, look for light red, finely textured meat. The bones should be reddish and moist, and any fat should be white, not yellow.
- Store cuts of lamb in the coldest part of the refrigerator for up to 3 days. If you won't be using the meat within 3 days, pop it in the freezer where chops and roasts will keep for 6 to 9 months.
- Ground lamb should be refrigerated and used or frozen within 24 hours. You can keep ground lamb in the freezer for 3 to 4 months.

Be a Fat Flush Cook

- Make lamb kebobs by placing bite size pieces of lamb on a skewer, along with your favorite Fat Flushing vegetables. Broil or grill and enjoy.
- Ground lamb makes delicious burgers. Season and cook as you would a hamburger.
- Braise lamb loin pieces in broth flavored with freshly minced garlic and a pinch of fennel.
- For a healthy twist on a traditional recipe, serve lamb with a mint yogurt sauce, which is made from plain yogurt, mint leaves, garlic, and cayenne.

SALMON

Fat Flush Factors

Energizer

Cholesterol Zapper

Blood-Sugar Stabilizer

The salmon is an amazing creature, traveling thousands of miles throughout its life cycle and returning, within 2 to 5 years, to spawn and die at the very location where it was born. There are six species of salmon, five in the Pacific Ocean and just one in the Atlantic. Their flesh ranges in color from pink to red to orange, with some varieties containing more health-giving omega-3 fatty acids than others. For example, chinook and sockeye salmon are fattier fish than pink and chum and contain abundant amounts of omega-3s.

Salmon is hugely popular around the world. An average portion provides over half the daily recommended allowance of energy-promoting protein while dishing up less saturated fat than an equal portion of any meat or poultry. These delicious fish also contain carotenoids (yellow and orange pigments that serve as antioxidants), vitamins A and D, and several B vitamins. However, in nutrition circles, it is the polyunsaturated fatty acids for which salmon is best known. These "good" fats help reduce the risk of heart disease, lower cholesterol, and slow the onset of inflammatory diseases. In fact, one study found that women who ate salmon on a weekly basis were 30 percent less likely to die of heart disease than women who ate fish only once a month.[3] Researchers have uncovered similar heart-healthy effects for men who eat fish regularly.

Remember, our bodies don't make essential fatty acids. It's up to us to provide them by eating the right kinds of foods. Studies have shown that about 60 percent of Americans are deficient in omega-3 essential fatty acids. So beef up your intake of omega-3s by putting salmon on your menu.

Recommended Usage: At least two servings of salmon per week.

Just the Facts

- Salmon is sold in many different forms. Fresh salmon comes whole or in steak or fillet form. You can also find frozen, canned, dried, or smoked salmon.

- Salmon may be wild or farm-raised. While both are rich in vitamins and essential fatty acids, you'll get the most nutritional value for your money with wild salmon.
- Norwegian salmon, a popular type of salmon often offered on restaurant menus, is actually Atlantic salmon that is farm-raised in Norway.

Boost the Benefits

- Fresh whole salmon should be displayed *buried* in ice, while fillets and steaks should be placed on top of the ice. Look for fish that is presented belly down so that the ice drains away from the fish as it melts. This reduces the chance of spoilage.
- If possible, smell salmon before buying it. Check for a mild "sea breeze" odor. If the fish smells like ammonia, it is definitely not fresh.
- Refrigerate salmon and prepare it within a day or two. Since most refrigerators are slightly warmer than ideal for storing fish, your best bet for maintaining freshness is to place salmon, tightly sealed in plastic wrap, in a baking dish filled with ice. Place the dish on the bottom shelf of the refrigerator and replenish the ice once or twice a day.
- You can prolong the shelf life of salmon by freezing it. Wrap it well in plastic and place it in the coldest part of the freezer where it should keep for about 2 to 3 weeks.
- If you buy commercially frozen salmon, check the package for signs of thawing such as lumps and ice crystals.
- Use frozen fish within 3 months. To thaw frozen fish, defrost it in the refrigerator. Do not refreeze it.
- If purchasing canned salmon, make sure it is packed in water, not oil. To get rid of excess sodium, drain the fish in a strainer, then rinse it under cold water.

Be a Fat Flush Cook

- If you notice a foamy white substance on the surface of salmon as you cook it, you may have overcooked the fish or prepared it at too high a temperature. The "white stuff" is a harmless protein, but you may want to modify your cooking technique next time.
- In general, whether you bake, poach, broil, or grill it, the cooking time for salmon is 10 minutes for every inch of thickness.
- To test for doneness, slip the point of a sharp knife into the thickest part of the fish and pull it aside. If flakes begin to separate, the fish is probably done and should be removed from the heat. Let it stand for three to four minutes to finish cooking.

- Use salmon in your favorite stir-fries, salads, soups, and even in Mexican dishes, such as tacos or burritos.
- Broil or grill salmon steaks and sprinkle them with dried mustard and flaxseed oil.
- Spruce up plain fish with lemon or lime juice and herbs such as dill, garlic, or parsley.
- For a yummy change of pace, try making a salmon burger—made with canned salmon in place of ground beef. Shape the fish into a patty and brown it in a non-stick skillet.

THINK TWICE!

- *Government inspection is not mandated for seafood, so buy your salmon from a reputable fish counter or market.*
- *While some fish are not considered safe for pregnant or nursing mothers or young children to eat, eating wild pacific salmon poses no safety concerns. At the seafood counter, ask for salmon marked as Alaskan salmon because it is guaranteed to be wild.*
- *Farm-raised salmon contains more contaminants than wild salmon because of overcrowding and exposure to feces.*

It's Been Said . . .

When making salmon for dinner, I always grill an extra portion and save it to use as a topping for my lunch salad the next day. This saves time and helps keep me on track with my weight loss.

JANE V., IOWA

WHEY PROTEIN

Fat Flush Factors

Energizer

Blood-Sugar Stabilizer

Cholesterol Zapper

Did you know that whey protein is the most easily absorbed, readily utilized protein, offering the most protein per serving? All that, and it's delicious, too! However, many people have never heard of whey protein, much less tasted it. Here's the scoop.

The two main proteins in milk are whey and casein. During the cheese-making process, these proteins are separated. The casein becomes cheese, and, until recently, the whey was disposed of down the drain or treated as "slop" for farm animals. But not anymore. Now we know the value of this nutritionally complete protein. Unlike soy or wheat protein, whey contains all the essential amino acids and has the highest number of branched chain amino acids (BCAA), which are crucial for a strong and healthy body.

Research has shown that consumption of whey helps reduce the risk of breast and colon cancer, hypertension, and heart disease. It boosts the immune system by increasing levels of glutathione, the most potent antioxidant in the body. Even dentists are pleased, since whey has been shown to reduce dental plaque and cavities.

In addition to increasing lean muscle mass and energizing the body, whey provides a number of other Fat Flushing benefits. It helps keep blood-sugar levels stable, which staves off the cravings that result from swings in your blood sugar. Components in whey help promote satiety by increasing the level of CCK, an appetite-suppressing hormone. Whey pumps up serotonin levels in the brain, which help fend off depression—and emotional eating.

The good news is that whey protein is easy and inexpensive to produce. But that's also the bad news. If you're not careful, you may end up with low-quality whey protein, which fails to produce the desired results. To maintain its integrity, whey protein must be processed under careful low-temperature and low-acid conditions. By checking the label for the term "whey protein isolates," you'll be assured of getting a high-quality product that has been processed properly.

To be considered a Fat Flushing superfood, whey protein must be compliant with the strictest Fat Flush criteria; it must be lactose-free, have no added sugar, and contain no artificial sweeteners. The only permissible sweetener is Stevia with inulin, a substance that nourishes the GI tract with friendly bacteria.

Recommended Usage: One or two servings of whey protein daily (depending on your activity level).

Just the Facts

- Whey's historical use as a medicinal food goes as far back as 400 B.C., to the time of Hippocrates.
- Because whey is so easily digested, it is a common ingredient in infant formulas and medically prescribed protein supplements.
- As the protein level of a whey protein increases, the amount of lactose it contains decreases.

Boost the Benefits

- Read the label carefully when buying whey protein. Whey protein *isolate* is the purest form of whey protein, containing between 90 to 95 percent protein and little to no fat or lactose. Whey protein *concentrate* is available in a number of different types based upon protein content, which can range between 25 to 89 percent.
- Be leery of buying whey protein out of a bulk bin. Inexpensive whey may be very low in protein and high in lactose. It may also have been cheaply processed at high temperatures, which reduces its nutritional value.
- Watch out, too, for hidden sugars or artificial sweeteners. Don't waste your money on whey protein that contains lactose, sugar, crystalline fructose, or artificial sweeteners such as aspartame, neotame, acesulfame K, sucralose, or Splenda. Do purchase whey protein that lists Stevia Plus or Stevia with inulin, a natural herbal product, as its only sweetener.

Be a Fat Flush Cook

- Whey protein can be mixed with water or juice to make a pleasant tasting and nutritious snack.
- Mix whey protein with your favorite frozen fruit and some cranberry juice. Add a dash of cinnamon, and you've got a terrific fat-burning meal or snack.

- Dissolve a bit of whey protein in water to make a substitute for cream in your herbal or organic coffee.
- Combine whey protein, water, and eggs to make a batter for crepe-like pancakes. Top them with your favorite fruit.

THINK TWICE!

Many people who have experienced lactose intolerance have no trouble consuming whey protein, especially if they select a pure whey protein isolate.

It's Been Said . . .

What would I do without my whey protein smoothies? I used to skip breakfast, but now I have a Fat Flushing whey smoothie every morning. It keeps me satisfied for hours, and I've dropped ten pounds in three weeks!

BECKY Z., CALIFORNIA

CHAPTER

3 Fat Flushing Vegetables

When diet is wrong, medicine is of no use.
When diet is correct, medicine is of no need.

ANCIENT AYURVEDIC PROVERB

"Finish your vegetables!" Didn't we all hear those words during our childhood years? Little did we know that it was some of the best advice we'd receive in our entire lives. Study after study has confirmed that people who eat more vegetables than other folks have a lower risk of developing chronic diseases and stand a good chance of maintaining a high quality of life well into their senior years.

From asparagus to zucchini, vegetables offer us a wealth of vitamins, fiber, and minerals, all of which are necessary for our wellbeing. Because our bodies can't stockpile these nutrients, we need to eat a variety of vegetables every day to ensure optimal health. A recent study by the National Cancer Institute found that Americans are indeed eating more vegetables than they did 25 years ago. Sadly, at least one fourth of those additional vegetables are French fries.[1]

Obviously, you won't find fried potatoes among the Fat Flushing vegetables in this chapter. However, you will find a delicious assortment of Mother Nature's bounty—vegetables that will help you maintain a healthy weight, reduce your risk of heart disease and diabetes, and offer protection against cancer. By decorating your dinner plate with a rainbow of vegetables, you'll fortify your body with the colorful pigments that give vegetables their antioxidant, disease-fighting power. In total, plant foods contain over 5000 antioxidants, including broccoli's *sulforaphane,* cabbage's *flavonoids,* and tomato's *lycopene,* all of which help protect the heart and stave off aging.

The 11 vegetables discussed in this chapter were chosen because they are Fat Flushing superfoods and provide a healthy balance of green, orange, and red "pigment power." If you mix and max these nutritious plant foods and eat generous daily portions as detailed in the Fat Flush Plan, you'll begin to notice a number of exciting side effects. Water retention will be a thing of the past; your cellulite will start to disappear; your skin will take on a healthy glow; and those snug clothes in your closet will suddenly fit like a glove!

ASPARAGUS

Fat Flush Factors

Diuretic

Detoxifier

First cultivated in Greece about 2500 years ago, asparagus offers a delicate, Fat Flushing flavor and tender texture. Originally, asparagus was used by ancient Greeks and Romans to relieve toothaches and prevent bee stings, but today it is well known as a diuretic. This vegetable's ability to fight water retention comes from the fact that it is high in potassium and low in sodium and contains an amino acid called *asparagine*. This trio also helps prevent fatigue by neutralizing ammonia, a substance that can build up in our bodies during the digestive process.

While asparagus may be considered a luxury vegetable, it pays for itself in nutritional benefits. Asparagus contains a special carbohydrate called *inulin* that is not digested but that helps feed the friendly bacteria in the large intestine. When we consume inulin regularly, these friendly bacteria proliferate, keeping the intestinal tract clear of unfriendly bacteria. In addition, asparagus is an excellent source of *glutathione*, an important anticarcinogen, and *rutin*, a substance that protects small blood vessels from rupturing.

There's more good news. Asparagus provides vitamins A and C, potassium, phosphorus, and iron. It's also a good source of fiber, the B-complex vitamins, and zinc. These delicate spears are also high in folic acid, which has been shown to reduce the risk of heart disease. Researchers believe that consuming 400 mcg of folic acid per day would decrease the heart attack rate in the United States by 10 percent.[2] Just one serving of asparagus provides over half of this recommended amount.

Recommended Usage: At least one 1/2 cup to 1 cup serving of asparagus per week.

Just the Facts

- Asparagus is a member of the lily family. While there are approximately 300 varieties of asparagus, only 20 of them are edible.

- Female asparagus stalks are plumper than male stalks and can grow as much as 10 inches in one day.
- The color of an asparagus spear, not its thickness, determines how tender it will be. Deep green or pure white spears are usually the most tender.
- White asparagus is not a different variety from the traditional green; it is simply grown in darkness. Green asparagus has a higher vitamin content than the white.

Boost the Benefits

- When you're shopping, look for straight asparagus stalks with firm stems of equal thickness. The tips should be tight, come to a point, and be deep green or purplish in color. Partially open or wilted tips are a hint that the asparagus is past its prime. Avoid asparagus that is excessively dirty or sandy.
- To ensure freshness, select asparagus that has been kept refrigerated or displayed upright in trays of cold water.
- The size of the stalk is not a measure of quality, but rather personal preference. While asparagus is usually found in bundles, you may see it sold loose. If so, select spears of the same size to ensure even cooking.
- To prevent rapid spoiling, always unband asparagus spears before storing them. Wrap the ends in a damp paper towel, place the spears in a plastic bag, and store the asparagus in your refrigerator.
- Since folate is destroyed by exposure to light, make a place in the *back* of the refrigerator for asparagus.
- While asparagus will keep for 4 or 5 days in the refrigerator, its flavor will diminish with each passing day. It's best to prepare and eat it the day you buy it.

Be a Fat Flush Cook

- When you're planning your menu, keep in mind that trimming and cooking causes asparagus to lose about half its total weight. A pound of asparagus serves two people as a main dish; three or four people as a side dish.
- Before cooking, snap off the tough bottom end of each asparagus stalk. But don't throw away those ends. Peel them and toss them in a pot of soup.
- You can buy a special asparagus steamer that holds the stalks upright while they cook. However, you may use any tall, lidded pot or a collapsible vegetable steamer placed in a large skillet.

- Cook asparagus *quickly*, or it becomes limp and discolored and takes on a bitter taste. Five to ten minutes should do the trick. To test for doneness, try to pierce the bottom of a stalk with the end of a paring knife. If the knife goes in, the asparagus is ready.
- For a different twist, add a clove of garlic, a slice of onion, or a lemon wedge to the water when you're cooking asparagus.
- After cooking, let asparagus spears drain on a paper towel for a minute before serving. If you plan to serve the asparagus cold, rinse it with cold water right away to stop the cooking process.
- Are you tired of plain scrambled eggs? Add a bit of chopped asparagus to give them color and flavor.

THINK TWICE

- *Cooking asparagus in a metal pan can cause discoloration of the metal.*
- *If you notice a strong odor to your urine after eating asparagus, don't panic. The harmless odor is caused by a chemical called* methyl mercaptan, *a by-product of the breakdown of asparagus.*

It's Been Said . . .

I marinate a pound of asparagus in 1/4 cup flax oil, 1 clove crushed garlic, 1 tsp fresh minced onion, 3 tbsp of lemon juice, and a dash of cayenne. After letting it stand for one hour, the asparagus is ready to eat or to chop and add to a tossed salad.

DEBRA F., CALIFORNIA

BROCCOLI

Fat Flush Factors

Cholesterol Zapper

Detoxifier

Blood-Sugar Stabilizer

A close relative of cauliflower, broccoli has been part of the American diet for over 200 years. Yet it wasn't until a 1930s radio campaign championing the benefits of broccoli that the public really caught on to this highly nutritious vegetable. Not only does broccoli provide a variety of textures, from soft to crunchy, but it also hits the jackpot as a Fat Flushing food. Iron, vitamin C, potassium, fiber—broccoli has all these and more! Munching on broccoli gives you abundant amounts of folic acid, calcium, and vitamin A.

Like other cruciferous vegetables, broccoli gives a boost to certain enzymes that help detoxify the body. Detoxification contributes to weight loss while helping to prevent cancer, diabetes, heart disease, osteoporosis, and high blood pressure. Worried about your cholesterol? Broccoli is known to contain a certain *pectin fiber* that binds to bile acids and keeps cholesterol from being released into the bloodstream. Does diabetes run in your family? At the USDA's Human Research Laboratory, a diabetes expert found that the chromium in broccoli may be effective in preventing type-2 diabetes by maintaining stable blood-sugar levels.[3]

In other research, at Johns Hopkins University, *sulforaphane*, a chemical found in broccoli, was found to kill H. pylori, bacteria that cause stomach ulcers and stomach cancers.[4] Sulforaphane even destroyed those strains of the bacteria that had become resistant to antibiotics. Broccoli is also a good source of folic acid, which scientists now believe serves as a defense against Alzheimer's disease. In addition, broccoli has been singled out as one of the few vegetables that significantly reduces the risk of heart disease.

How's that for a deal? For just pennies per serving, broccoli serves up a feast of Fat Flushing properties and helps keep you lean, strong, and healthy!

Recommended Usage: At least 3 to 5 cups of broccoli per week.

Just the Facts

- "Broccoli" comes from the Latin word "brachium," which means strong arm or branch.
- Some broccoli hybrids include *broccolini*, a cross between broccoli and Chinese kale; *broccoflower*, a cross between broccoli and cauliflower; and *purple broccoli*, a cousin of broccoli, which looks like small heads of purple cauliflower.
- Ounce for ounce, broccoli offers more vitamin C than an orange and as much calcium as a glass of milk. One medium spear has three times more fiber than a slice of wheat bran bread and over 1000 IUs of vitamin A.
- Broccoli sprouts are tiny 3-day-old plants that resemble alfalfa sprouts and have a peppery flavor. Researchers estimate that, depending on their age, broccoli sprouts contain up to 100 times the nutritional power of mature broccoli.
- A typical bunch of broccoli weighs about 2 pounds, which is enough to serve as a side dish for three or four people.

Boost the Benefits

- You can rely on the color of broccoli to serve as an indicator of its nutritional value. Florets that are dark green, purplish, or bluish green contain more beta-carotene and vitamin C than paler florets. Select broccoli with compact floret clusters that are uniform in color.
- Bypass broccoli that is bruised or yellowed or that has a brown or slimy stalk. And, if you see yellow flowers beginning to blossom within the clusters, the broccoli is overripe and will be tough and woody—no matter how you cook it.
- Fresh broccoli has a clean "green" smell, so, if you notice a strong odor, the broccoli is past its prime.
- Fresh broccoli is at its best if it is used within a day or two of purchase, but it will keep for up to 4 days if stored in your refrigerator's crisper. Alternately, you can stand broccoli up, bouquet style, in a jar of water, cover it with a plastic bag, and store it on a shelf in the fridge.
- If you have an abundance of broccoli, don't let it go bad. Instead, blanch it, and then pop it in the freezer where it will keep for up to 1 year.

Be a Fat Flush Cook

- Very fresh, young broccoli is tender enough to be served raw or tossed in a salad.

- Do you throw away broccoli leaves? If so, you're discarding the highest concentration of beta-carotene. The leaves are edible, so try adding them to your salad greens.
- Cooked broccoli should be tender enough so that you can pierce the stalks with a sharp knife, but it should still be crisp and bright. To ensure that the stalks cook as quickly as the florets, cut an X in the bottom of each stalk and/or a lengthwise slit in the stems.
- Sprinkle lemon juice and ground flaxseeds over lightly steamed broccoli.
- Chop some broccoli, and add it to your morning omelet.

THINK TWICE!

- *Like its cruciferous relatives, broccoli contains goitrogens, naturally occurring substances that can interfere with thyroid function. If you have been diagnosed with a thyroid disorder, you may want to check with your physician before you consume large amounts of broccoli.*
- *Keep in mind that packaged, frozen broccoli contains twice as much sodium and fewer health-promoting phytochemicals as fresh broccoli.*

Fat Flush Fun

Do not let the smell of the sulfur compounds released while broccoli is cooking keep you away from this nutritious vegetable. Drop a large piece of stale bread in the cooking water to counteract the odor.

It's Been Said . . .

I have found that the Fat Flushing herbs and spices that go best with broccoli include dill, mustard seed, cayenne, and garlic.

DIANE L., NEW YORK

I do not like broccoli. And I haven't liked it since I was a little kid and my mother made me eat it. And I'm President of the United States and I'm not going to eat any more broccoli.

GEORGE BUSH, U.S. PRESIDENT, 1990

CABBAGE

Fat Flush Factor

Detoxifier

One of the world's oldest vegetables, cabbage continues to be an inexpensive dietary staple. Because it is easy to grow, we are lucky enough to find this nutritional powerhouse throughout the year, although it is at its best during the late fall and winter.

A member of the cruciferous family, which includes broccoli and kale, cabbage is rich in cancer-fighting nutrients, including Vitamin C, fiber, and two phytochemicals, sulforaphane and indoles. These two compounds help detoxify the body, ridding it of cancer-producing substances, including excess estrogen. A number of studies have shown that women who include cabbage regularly in their diet reduce their risk of breast cancer by 45 percent.

Cabbage has powerful antibacterial properties as well. Decades ago, researchers at Stanford University determined that consuming cabbage is a good treatment for peptic ulcers.[5] Glutamine is an amino acid that nourishes the cells that line the stomach and small intestine. The high glutamine content of cabbage allows it to heal ulcers, often in as few as 10 days. So, if your consumption of cabbage has been limited to coleslaw or sauerkraut, take another look at this fantastic Fat Flushing vegetable.

Recommended Usage: At least three 1/2 cup to 1 cup servings of cabbage per week.

Just the Facts

- There are at least a hundred different types of cabbage grown throughout the world, but the most common types in the United States are the green, red, and Savoy varieties. Both green and red cabbages have smooth textured leaves, while Savoy leaves are ruffled.
- The outer cabbage leaves are darker and contain more nutrients than the pale inner leaves, which develop without the benefit of sunlight.

Boost the Benefits

- Buy solid, heavy cabbage heads with shiny, crisp, colorful leaves. Watch out for cracks, bruises, and blemishes because damage to the outer leaves suggests hidden worm damage or decay.

- If there are no outer leaves on the cabbage, it means that the head has already been trimmed and may well have come from storage rather than from a fresh harvest.
- Once cabbage is cut, it loses its vitamin C content rapidly. So, while buying precut cabbage may be convenient, it will cost you important nutrients.
- Keeping cabbage cold keeps it fresh and helps retain its vitamin C content. Place the whole head in a perforated plastic bag in the crisper of your refrigerator where it will stay fresh for about 2 weeks.
- Once the head has been cut, place the remainder in a plastic bag in the refrigerator. Your best bet is to use it up in a day or two.
- Because phytonutrients in the cabbage react with carbon steel, turning the leaves black, cut it with a stainless steel knife.

Be a Fat Flush Cook

- Cut up fresh cabbage and sprinkle it with lemon, and you've got a delicious afternoon snack.
- Throw in some chopped cabbage when making vegetable soup.
- Toss shredded red and white cabbage with fresh lemon juice and a bit of flaxseed or olive oil. Spice it up with some turmeric, cumin, coriander, and cayenne to make colorful coleslaw with a Fat Flush twist.
- Use cabbage leaves as a wrapper for cooked meats or veggies.
- Steam some sliced cabbage and top it with your favorite spaghetti sauce.
- Top a chicken sandwich with some shredded cabbage.

It's Been Said . . .

For a filling Fat Flush side dish, I like to combine some red cabbage with a chopped apple. I simmer it in some salt-free vegetable broth, and it's ready to serve in minutes!

Wendy W., Oregon

The cabbage surpasses all other vegetables. If, at a banquet, you wish to dine a lot and enjoy your dinner, then eat as much cabbage as you wish, seasoned with vinegar, before dinner, and likewise after dinner eat some half-dozen leaves. It will make you feel as if you had not eaten, and you can drink as much as you like.

Marcus Porcius Cato (Roman politician, 234–149 B.C.)

CAULIFLOWER

Fat Flush Factor

Detoxifier

Originating in ancient Asia, cauliflower is in the same cruciferous family as broccoli, kale, cabbage, and collards. However, because its heavy green leaves shield the flowering head from the sun, cauliflower lacks the green chlorophyll found in its "cousins." Instead, it remains milky white, with a spongy texture and sweet, slightly nutty flavor.

Cauliflower contains a high amount of vitamin C, folate, fiber, and complex carbohydrates. As a cruciferous vegetable, cauliflower has been studied for its role in reducing the risk of cancer. Scientists know that, for people with cancer, it is essential to rapidly detoxify toxins in the liver before they have a chance to encourage cell deregulation and uncontrolled cancerous growth. Cauliflower contains both glucosinolates and thiocyanates, compounds that increase the liver's ability to neutralize potential toxins. There are a number of enzymes in cauliflower, such as glutathione transferase, that also help with the detoxifying process.

Detoxification is also essential to weight loss and general health, so give cauliflower a prominent spot on your Fat Flushing menu.

Recommended Usage: At least 3 cups of cauliflower per week.

Just the Facts

- The compact head of a cauliflower is called a "curd" and is composed of undeveloped flower buds.
- A medium-sized cauliflower head, measuring 6 inches in diameter and weighing about 2 pounds, will serve four people.

Boost the Benefits

- When shopping for cauliflower, look for creamy white heads that are firm, compact, and heavy for their size. Just say no to cauliflower with brown patches or spots.
- You'll get a fresher head of cauliflower if it is protected by a number of thick leaves. Should you pick a small or large cauliflower?

Size does not affect taste or quality, so go with the one that suits your needs.

- Buying precut cauliflower florets is probably not the best choice because they will lose their freshness after a day or two.
- If refrigerated in a perforated plastic bag, uncooked cauliflower will keep for up to a week. To prevent moisture from settling in the floret clusters, store the head with the leaves still on and the stem side down.
- Cooked cauliflower spoils faster, so don't store it in the refrigerator longer than a day or two.

Be a Fat Flush Cook

- When heated, cauliflower releases a sulfurlike odor that some people find unpleasant. The longer you cook cauliflower, the stronger the odor. So, to minimize the smell—and preserve the nutrients—cook cauliflower for only a short time.
- Cauliflower may turn yellow if it is prepared in alkaline water. For whiter cauliflower, add a tablespoon or two of lemon juice to the cooking water.
- Don't waste those cauliflower stems and leaves. They are terrific for adding to soup stocks.
- For creating cauliflower with a surprising yellow color, boil it briefly with a spoonful of turmeric.
- Simmer cauliflower florets in a bit of broth with freshly minced garlic and ginger.
- For a quick soup, puree cooked cauliflower; add fennel seeds and your other favorite Fat Flushing herbs and spices. Serve hot or cold.
- Don't forget that raw cauliflower makes a great, portable snack. It also adds texture and taste to your favorite tossed salad.
- Add chopped cauliflower florets to your favorite pasta sauce.

THINK TWICE!

- *If you have been diagnosed with a thyroid condition, you may want to stick to cooked cauliflower. Cooking inactivates the goitrogenic compounds found in cauliflower. These substances occur naturally in certain foods and can interfere with thyroid function.*
- *Do not cook cauliflower in an aluminum or iron pot. Aluminum reacts with the phytochemicals in cauliflower and causes the florets to turn yellow, while iron causes cauliflower to take on a brownish or blue-green hue.*

It's Been Said . . .

I've never left the table hungry when mashed cauliflower is part of my meal. And it's so easy to prepare! Just steam some cauliflower, mash with a bit of broth and your favorite herbs . . . and voila! You've got a terrific Fat Flushing substitute for mashed potatoes.

KARI W., ILLINOIS

Cauliflower is nothing but cabbage with a college education.

MARK TWAIN

CUCUMBERS

Fat Flush Factor

Diuretic

Originating in Asia over 10,000 years ago, cucumbers are grown for slicing or pickling. Slicing, or "table" cucumbers, are cylindrical in shape and usually range in length from 6 to 9 inches, while pickling "cukes" are smaller. If you see a foot-long cucumber, it is probably an English or hothouse variety.

The pale green flesh of a cucumber is mostly water, making it a moist and cooling treat. This fresh-tasting veggie adds crunch and fiber to any meal, while offering plenty of vitamin C, silica, potassium, and magnesium. A cucumber's vitamin C content helps calm irritated skin and reduce swelling, which is why cucumber slices are used at expensive spas to soothe tired, puffy eyes.

However, cucumbers do more than give a glow to your skin. Since silica is an essential component of healthy connective tissue, cucumbers help build strong muscles, tendons, and bones. Studies have shown that the minerals in cucumbers can fight hypertension by reducing systolic blood pressure by at least 5 points. And a generous helping of Fat Flushing cucumber works to hydrate the body and reduce excess water weight.

Recommended Usage: One cucumber daily.

Just the Facts

- Because a cucumber is 95 percent water, its inside can be up to 20 degrees cooler than its outside temperature.
- Technically, the cucumber is a fruit and is related to the watermelon.
- Columbus brought the first cucumber seed to America.
- While cucumber seeds are edible, some people find the seedless English cucumber easier to digest.

Boost the Benefits

- Look for cucumbers with smooth, bright skin and an even green color. They should be firm, with no withered or shriveled ends.

Steer clear of cucumbers that are yellow or that have sunken areas.

- Size does matter! In general, smaller cucumbers have a sweeter taste and fewer seeds than larger cucumbers.
- If you refrigerate cucumbers quickly after purchase, they should keep for about 1 week. However, since they are sensitive to temperature extremes, place your cucumbers close to the top of the fridge, which is often warmer. Storing them in a paper or cloth bag will keep them from catching a "chill."
- Most cucumbers are waxed to protect them from bruising during shipping. If you buy waxed cucumbers, be sure to peel them before you eat them. You'll save time, nutrients, *and* color by selecting unwaxed cucumbers, which may be eaten with the skin on. Organic cucumbers are a good choice, as are English cucumbers which are wrapped in plastic.
- If cucumbers are exposed to weather extremes as they grow, they can develop a bitter taste. If you come across a bitter cucumber, discard an inch or so from the stem end, remove the seeds, and peel the entire cucumber. This should get rid of most of the harsh flavor.
- To seed a cucumber, peel it and cut it in half lengthwise. With the tip of a spoon or a melon baller, scrape the center from top to bottom to scoop out the seeds from each half.

Be a Fat Flush Cook

- Serving suggestion: Often, cucumbers straight out of the fridge are too cold to eat comfortably. Consider taking them out of the fridge when you first begin your meal preparation.
- Are you looking for a quick and easy snack? Slice a cucumber and enjoy it raw.
- Add sliced cucumber to your tossed salads.
- Forget the second piece of bread. Top your sandwiches with crispy cucumber slices instead.
- Cook sliced cucumbers with your favorite Fat Flushing herbs.
- For a tasty side dish, combine cucumber slices with thinly sliced red onion, plain yogurt, and fresh dill.
- Add diced cucumber to tuna fish or chicken salad recipes.

THINK TWICE!

- *Cucumbers can cause an unpleasant mouth itch in people who are allergic to pollen or aspirin.*

- *The wax used on cucumbers may be a plant, insect, animal, or petroleum-based product. To avoid problems with these "unknown" substances, choose organic cucumbers.*

It's Been Said . . .

One of my favorite salads is a mixture of diced cucumbers with snow peas, tossed with some flax oil and apple cider vinegar. I add some fresh parsley and a dash of cayenne.

VICKY S., TEXAS

JÍCAMA

Fat Flush Factor

Cholesterol Zapper

Like many other Fat Flushers, I find jícama to be a cross between a potato and an apple—with a bit of water chestnut thrown in for good measure. This large, bulbous root is a popular Mexican vegetable with a sweet flavor and crunchy texture. Because jícama can be used either raw or cooked, it is a very versatile vegetable. Even cooked, it retains its crisp, water chestnut type of texture and flavor.

With its increasing popularity across the America, more and more supermarkets are carrying jícama. Look for a brownish gray root vegetable, shaped something like a turnip—or ask the produce manager to point you in the right direction. Extremely nutritious, jícama is low in sodium and contains no fat, making it a dieter's delight. A cup of jícama provides nearly 6 grams of fiber, which help to satisfy the appetite and aid the digestive process. In addition, jícama is bursting with vitamin C. One of vitamin C's important functions is to keep LDL cholesterol from oxidizing—for only cholesterol that has been damaged by oxidation causes heart disease. Vitamin C may also protect against heart disease by "relaxing" stiff arteries and preventing platelets from clumping together.

As jícama becomes better known throughout kitchens in America, it will continue to show up in salads and stir-fries everywhere. If you haven't yet tried this unusual vegetable, give it a whirl. No doubt, you will enjoy it as much as I do.

Recommended Usage: 1 cup daily, or as desired.

Just the Facts

- You may hear jícama called a yam bean, Mexican potato, or Chinese turnip.
- Jícama is pronounced "HEE-kuh-muh."
- Raw jícama tastes something like a nice crisp apple or pear.
- "Arrowroot," a common cooking thickener, is made from jícama.

Boost the Benefits

- At the store, look for a firm, heavy jícama that has smooth, relatively unblemished skin.
- While jícama can weigh up to 6 pounds, the smaller roots, weighing 3 pounds or less, offer better flavor and more juice than the larger ones.
- Store a whole jícama in a cool, dry place, because too much moisture can cause mold. It should stay fresh for up to 2 weeks.
- To avoid discoloration of the flesh, wash and peel jícama just before using it.
- Once you cut into the jícama, wrap any cut pieces in plastic and refrigerate them. It should maintain its freshness and flavor for 1 week.

Be a Fat Flush Cook

- Sliced or grated jícama adds a crunchy texture to any salad or slaw.
- For a delicious snack, try cutting jícama into cubes and mixing them with lime juice and a dusting of cayenne.
- Jícama may also be baked, boiled, or mashed like potatoes.
- When jícama is combined with other foods, it tends to take on the flavors of those ingredients. This ability to blend with other vegetables and seasonings makes jícama a lovely complement to stir-fry dishes.
- If you substitute jícama for water chestnuts in any recipe, you'll save some pennies!

It's Been Said . . .

I've dropped fifteen pounds in two months of Fat Flushing and jícama has really helped. I eat it every day as an afternoon snack. Sometimes I eat it plain; other times I spice it up with cayenne or cinnamon. It satisfies my urge to crunch . . . and has taken the place of potato chips in my life!

MARY F., KANSAS

KALE

Fat Flush Factors

Detoxifier

Energizer

Cholesterol Zapper

Blood-Sugar Stabilizer

One of the top vegetable sources of vitamin A, kale is a leafy green vegetable that belongs to the same family as cabbage, collards, and Brussels sprouts. In fact, kale is known as the "grandmother" of the entire cabbage family. Kale resembles collards, except that its leaves are curly at the edges. When cooked, kale shrinks less than other greens and offers a stronger flavor and coarser texture. Your local grocer probably carries the deep green variety, but kale also comes in yellow-green, red, or purple, with either flat or ruffled leaves.

Kale provides more nutritional value for fewer calories than almost any other food. A cup of kale serves up an abundance of manganese, a trace mineral that helps produce energy from protein and carbohydrates. Manganese is also a critical component of an essential antioxidant enzyme called *superoxide dismutase,* which provides important protection against free radicals. Kale supplies both vitamin B^6 and riboflavin, a dynamic duo that protects lipids like cholesterol from being attacked—and damaged—by free radicals. The high fiber content of kale helps reduce cholesterol levels and keep blood-sugar levels under control.

As a Fat Flushing food, kale offers calcium for healthy bones, lutein to protect the eyes from cataracts, indole-3-carbinol to guard against colon cancer, plus a healthy dose of iron, vitamin A, and vitamin C. Do yourself a favor by grabbing a supply of these superstar greens next time you go shopping.

Recommended Usage: Daily, as desired.

Just the Facts

- Kale is available year-round, but it is most tender and flavorful during the winter months.

- You may substitute kale for spinach in just about any recipe you like.
- One cup of kale provides over 200 percent more than the daily requirement of vitamin A and 75 percent of the daily need for vitamin C.
- While edible, colored varieties of kale, sometimes called *salad savoy*, are most often grown for ornamental purposes. They do have a stronger flavor than regular kale.

Boost the Benefits

- Look for crisp, dark, bluish-green leaves that are not wilted, yellowing, or marked by tiny holes. The stems, which are edible, should be plump and moist.
- If you see kale with smaller-sized leaves, grab it up because it is especially tender and offers a mild flavor. Coarse, over-sized leaves are likely to be tough and bitter.
- To store kale, wrap it in a damp paper towel, place it in a perforated plastic bag and keep it in the coldest part of the refrigerator. Washing it before you store it may cause it to become limp.
- Kale can be kept in the refrigerator for several days, although it is best when eaten within a day or two, since the longer it is stored, the stronger its flavor becomes. Even if the leaves still look nice and green, they will have an unpleasant taste after a day or two.
- To remove the sand and dirt from kale, wash it prior to cooking by swishing the separate leaves in a large basin of cool water. Lift the leaves from the water, let the sand and grit settle to the bottom, and repeat if necessary. Do not soak the leaves.

Be a Fat Flush Cook

- If the kale stems are thin and tender, just trim off the very tips and cook the stems along with the leaves. If the stems are tough, remove them by folding each leaf in half, vein-side out, and pulling up on the stem as you keep the leaf folded.
- You may use whole kale leaves if they are small, but it's best to strip larger leaves from the center rib. To shred kale, place the leaves in a pile, roll them up together, and cut them into thin slices.
- Baby kale may be eaten raw and is delicious mixed with other greens in a salad.
- Mature kale is too tough to consume raw. You may steam, blanch, braise, sauté, or boil it. Depending on the method, cooking time varies from 5 to 30 minutes.

- Whenever possible, plan to use the cooking liquid from kale in a sauce or soup broth so that none of the nutrients are wasted.
- Try adding chopped kale to soups and stews.
- Braise chopped kale and apples. Before serving, sprinkle with apple cider vinegar and slivered almonds.

THINK TWICE!

Kale is among a small number of foods that contain oxalates, naturally occurring substances that can crystallize in the body and cause kidney stones. If you have been diagnosed with kidney or gallbladder problems, check with your physician before making kale a frequent menu item.

It's Been Said . . .

A huge serving of kale on my plate really fills me up and helps me maintain my thirty pound weight loss. I love to sauté it in broth with some fresh garlic. Just before serving, I sprinkle it with some lemon juice and a dash of olive oil.

MAGGIE T., VERMONT

SPAGHETTI SQUASH

Fat Flush Factors

Cholesterol Zapper

Blood-Sugar Stabilizer

What vegetable looks like a small, yellow watermelon and can take the place of pasta at dinner? It's spaghetti squash, a variety of winter squash with mildly sweet flesh that pulls apart to form slender spaghettilike strands. Averaging from 4 to 8 pounds each, spaghetti squash can usually be found year-round and offers a bounty of nutritional benefits.

While research is ongoing, preliminary studies have shown that juice from squash has the ability to assist the body in fighting both cancerlike cell mutations and prostate problems. Beta-carotene, one of the most abundant nutrients in spaghetti squash, has powerful antioxidant and anti-inflammatory properties. It can prevent the oxidation of cholesterol in the body, regulate blood-sugar levels, and thwart insulin resistance. The potassium found in spaghetti squash helps to lower blood pressure, and its fiber keeps cancer-causing chemicals from attacking colon cells.

As an added bonus, spaghetti squash is an excellent source of folate, which is needed by the body to break down a dangerous metabolic by-product called *homocysteine*. Since homocysteine can damage blood vessel walls, consuming plenty of folate can decrease your risk for heart attack and stroke. So, while spaghetti squash has a hard shell that can be quite difficult to pierce, it is definitely worth the trouble.

Recommended Usage: At least 1 cup of spaghetti squash per week.

Just the Facts

- Vegetable spaghetti, vegetable marrow, spaghetti squash, noodle squash, and squaghetti are all names for this versatile vegetable.
- You'll end up with about 5 cups of "spaghetti" from the average 4-pound squash.
- A spaghetti squash with a soft rind may be watery and lacking in flavor.

- Spaghetti squash with a dark, orange color has more beta-carotene than squashes with pale flesh.

Boost the Benefits

- At the store, look for a firm squash that is heavy for its size. The rind should have a dull sheen and a pale, even color. If the stem is still attached, it should be dry and rounded, not moist, shriveled, or blackened.
- Soft spots and green color are signs that the squash is not ripe. Moldy, water-soaked areas are indications of decay.
- Do not wash winter squash before storing it. Spaghetti squash can be stored at room temperature for about a month, but once you've cut into it, it will keep in the refrigerator for up to 2 days.
- Spaghetti squash freezes well. Pack cooked squash into freezer bags and toss them into the freezer. Before using, thaw the squash partially, and then steam for about 5 minutes.

Be a Fat Flush Cook

- If you have trouble cutting through the shell of a spaghetti squash, try cooking it in a slow cooker. Select a squash that fits into your slow cooker. Pierce it several times with a large fork or skewer. Place it in the slow cooker and add 2 cups of water. Cover and cook on low for 8 to 9 hours. Cut in half and enjoy.
- Spaghetti squash can also be baked, boiled or steamed. Once the squash is cooked, let it cool for 10 minutes before cutting it in half. Remove the seeds and pull a fork lengthwise through the flesh to separate it into long strands.
- Serve spaghetti squash with your favorite pasta sauce.
- Chill the squash strands, and then toss them with your favorite Fat Flush dressing. Add some fresh tomato chunks, and you've got a refreshing—and beautiful—side dish.

It's Been Said . . .

A great idea for leftover spaghetti squash is to mix in an egg, add whatever herbs and spices you like, ladle the mixture (by the 1/4 cupful) into a hot skillet (coated with a quick spray of olive oil), and cook like pancakes. You can make this savory or sweet . . . my family loves theirs with cinnamon and Stevia.

LINDA S., FLORIDA

TOMATOES

Fat Flush Factors

Cholesterol Zapper

Blood-Sugar Stabilizer

Energizer

A century ago, most Americans considered the tomato to be an odd, even poisonous, food. How times have changed. Today, sweet, juicy tomatoes are a staple in homes—and gardens—all across the United States. Tomatoes come in many different varieties. In addition to the "basic" tomato, your local grocery may carry petite cherry tomatoes, bright yellow tomatoes, Italian pear-shaped tomatoes, and the small green tomato, or tomatillo, common in Mexican fare.

Tomatoes are an excellent source of vitamins C and A, providing detoxifying antioxidants to neutralize dangerous free radicals that could otherwise damage cells and escalate problems with atherosclerosis, diabetic complications, asthma, and colon cancer. In addition, tomatoes supply fiber, which has been shown to lower cholesterol levels, control blood-sugar levels, and help prevent colon cancer.

Tomatoes offer a trio of notable heart-healthy nutrients: potassium, vitamin B^6, and folate. In addition, studies in the U.S. and Europe have concluded that lycopene, a phytonutrient found in tomatoes, lowers cholesterol levels and reduces the risk of heart disease.[6] Tomatoes improve your body's energy production by supplying a bounty of biotin and help maintain bone health by serving as a source of vitamin K. And those blood-sugar levels, already supported by the fiber in tomatoes, are stabilized even further by their chromium content.

Tomatoes are a marvelous vegetable loaded with an array of critical nutrients. By increasing your consumption of tomatoes, you'll take a big step forward toward flushing your fat and improving your health.

Recommended Usage: Daily, as desired.

Just the Facts

- Although technically a fruit, tomatoes can't pass for dessert the way other fruits can. Their sweetness is subtle, toned down by a high acid content and slightly bitter flavor.

- The most concentrated source of vitamin C in a tomato is the jelly-like substance surrounding the seeds. But keep in mind that a hothouse-grown tomato has half the vitamin C content of a vine-ripened tomato.
- In France, the tomato is called a *pomme d'amour*, or "love apple," since it is believed to be an aphrodisiac.
- Combining tomatoes with bread or other starches creates an acidic reaction in the body, causing an upset stomach in some people. To avoid this, eat tomatoes alone or with other fresh vegetables.

Boost the Benefits

- Look for well-shaped, smooth tomatoes with no wrinkles, cracks, bruises, or soft spots. For the best flavor, select tomatoes with a deep, rich color. The deep color indicates that the fruit is loaded with the desirable antioxidant, lycopene.
- Take a pass on puffy-looking tomatoes because they tend to be watery.
- Generally, the best tasting tomatoes are the ones grown locally because they have been allowed to mature and ripen on the vine. Most local tomatoes contain twice as much vitamin C as tomatoes that were picked green or grown in a hothouse. Use your nose to check for a vine-ripened tomato. It should have a fresh, tomato smell, while a tomato that was picked green and then ripened artificially has a "gassy" or chemical smell.
- Store tomatoes at room temperature, away from direct sunlight. They will keep for up to a week, depending upon how ripe they are when they are purchased.
- To speed up the ripening process, place tomatoes in a paper bag, along with an apple. The ethylene gas emitted by the apple will help mature the tomatoes.
- If the tomatoes ripen but you are not yet ready to eat them, place them in the refrigerator, where they will keep for a day or two. Remove them from the refrigerator about an hour before using them to allow for maximum flavor and juiciness.
- Whole tomatoes, chopped tomatoes, and tomato sauce freeze well, so don't be afraid to stock up when you find vine-ripened tomatoes.
- To get the greatest health benefits from the nutrients and the fiber, eat your tomatoes unpeeled.

Be a Fat Flush Cook

- If your recipe requires *seeded* tomatoes, cut the fruit in half horizontally and gently scoop the seeds out with a teaspoon.
- Add chopped tomatoes to your favorite vegetable soup recipe.

- Combine chopped onions, tomatoes, cumin, and cayenne for a super easy salsa.
- Instead of a second piece of bread, top your sandwich with a couple of deep red tomato slices.
- To prevent tomatoes from turning acidic, simmer them slowly rather than bringing them to a rolling boil.

THINK TWICE!

- *If you purchase canned tomatoes, check the label to make sure they were produced in the United States. Many foreign countries do not have high standards for lead content in cans. The high acid content of tomatoes can cause lead to leech into the can's contents.*
- *Avoid aluminum cookware when preparing tomatoes since their high acid content interacts with aluminum and may cause metal to leach into the food.*
- *If you hit a plateau when dieting, consider cutting down on your consumption of tomatoes. They rate a 25 on the glycemic index, while most of the other Fat Flushing vegetables score less than 15. (The glycemic index ranks foods based on their immediate effect on your blood sugar. The lower the score, the less impact the food has on blood-sugar levels.)*

Fat Flush Fun

A small boy was looking at the red ripe tomatoes growing in the farmer's garden.

"I'll give you my two pennies for that tomato," said the boy pointing to a beautiful, large, ripe fruit hanging on the vine.

"No," said the farmer, *"I get a dime for a tomato like that one."*

The small boy pointed to a smaller green one.

"Will you take two pennies for that one?"

"Yes," replied the farmer, *"I'll give you that one for two cents."*

"OK," said the lad, sealing the deal by putting the coins in the farmer's hand, *"I'll pick it up in about a week."*

It's Been Said . . .

I make my own Fat Flush spaghetti sauce by sautéing some fresh garlic in beef broth, adding chopped tomatoes and seasoning with my favorite herbs and spices. I let the mixture simmer until it has a rich, deep flavor. Then, I serve it over spaghetti squash for a fabulous Fat Flushing meal!

JANET V., OKLAHOMA

WATERCRESS

Fat Flush Factors

Detoxifier

Diuretic

Watercress is the stuff legends are made of. According to Greek mythology, the god, Zeus, fortified himself against his enemies by eating watercress. In 460 B.C., Hippocrates located his hospital near a stream so he would have access to fresh watercress, his treatment of choice for many ailments. And, in nineteenth century England, street vendors sold bunches of watercress as a handheld treat, to be eaten like an ice cream cone! So why do most people view watercress as mere garnish—a touch of green to decorate the plate?

Perhaps it's the pungent flavor, which is reminiscent of mustard, but with a refreshing, rather than fiery "bite" that makes watercress something of an acquired taste. If you have yet to make the acquaintance of this Fat Flushing vegetable, consider adding it to your grocery list. Watercress is still grown using traditional gravel beds fed by fresh flowing spring water and contains a bounty of blood-purifying phytonutrients.

One such beneficial nutrient is the anticancer compound *phenylethyl isothiocyanate*, or PEITC. Whenever it is crushed, chopped, or chewed, watercress releases a peppery flavor, evidence of the PEITC content. The more pungent the taste, the more PEITC is being released, and the greater the health benefit.

In addition, watercress contains generous amounts of vitamins A and C, along with hefty doses of calcium, folic acid, potassium, and iron. Regular consumption of watercress boosts kidney efficiency and does away with hunger pangs. Best of all, watercress is a superb natural diuretic, serving as a powerful Fat Flushing tool for reducing water retention and bloating.

Recommended Usage: At least one bunch of watercress per week.

Just the Facts

- Watercress is a fantastic source of vitamin C and, ounce for ounce, contains more iron than spinach and more calcium than milk.

- Watercress can grow anywhere there is running water.
- The Chinese eat ten times more watercress than Americans do, often tossing two or three bunches into one stir-fried dish.

Boost the Benefits

- Look for glossy, dark green watercress leaves and crisp stems.
- Typically, young watercress contains less mustard oil than older watercress, but is easier to digest, allowing the body to get the most benefit from the phytonutrients.
- Watercress should be kept moist with damp paper towels, wrapped in plastic, and stored in the refrigerator. It will keep this way for about a week.
- If necessary, revitalize watercress by submerging it in ice water, discarding any wilted, bruised, or yellow leaves.

Be a Fat Flush Cook

- Use watercress like you would any lettuce, giving the stems a slight trim.
- Toss fresh watercress leaves into a mixture of Fat Flushing berries. Top with a squeeze of lemon juice for a delicious dessert idea.
- Watercress and ginger combine well in any stir-fry dish.
- Add chopped watercress to your next omelet.
- Cooking mellows the mustardy bite of watercress, making it a fantastic addition to any soup. You can also steam it as a side dish for fish or poultry.

It's Been Said . . .

My favorite sandwich is a piece of spelt bread, heaped with some sliced chicken breast and topped with plenty of watercress. Depending on my mood, I'll add some Fat Flush spices. My current favorite is cayenne.

MITCH P., COLORADO

The eating of watercress doth restore the wanted bloom to the cheeks of old-young ladies.

LORD FRANCIS BACON, ENGLISH PHILOSOPHER

ZUCCHINI

Fat Flush Factors

Cholesterol Zapper

Detoxifier

Probably the best known of the summer squashes, the zucchini is a cousin to both the melon and the cucumber. Native to America, it was brought back to Europe by Christopher Columbus. Today, zucchini is grown and enjoyed around the world, especially between May and July, when it is most abundant.

Zucchini's creamy white flesh has a delicate flavor, but the entire vegetable is edible and nutritious, including its flesh, skin, and seeds. Zucchini is a good source of vitamins A, B^6, and C and potassium, magnesium, folate, riboflavin, and fiber; many of these nutrients help prevent atherosclerosis and diabetic heart disease. The magnesium in zucchini reduces the risk of heart attack and stroke, while the potassium brings down high blood pressure. The vitamin C and beta-carotene found in zucchini helps prevent the oxidation of cholesterol, keeping atherosclerosis at bay. And zucchini's vitamin B^6 and folate are used to break down *homocysteine*, a substance that contributes to heart disease.

The nutrients in zucchini offer valuable protection against other diseases as well. The high fiber content of zucchini absorbs cancer-causing toxins, keeping them away from cells in the colon. The beta-carotene found in zucchini has anti-inflammatory properties that fight conditions such as asthma, arthritis, and irritable bowel syndrome. During your next trip to the supermarket, load up on these lean, green, disease-fighting veggies.

Recommended Usage: Daily, as desired.

Just the Facts

- Generally, one medium-sized zucchini serves one person.
- Zucchini is the most popular of the summer squashes and the only vegetable that begins with the letter *z*.

- The flavor of zucchini is sweetest when it is less than 6 inches long. Zucchinis can grow as large as baseball bats, but, when they reach this size, they have little flavor and large, tough seeds.

Boost the Benefits

- When you're shopping, look for zucchinis that are firm, glossy, and heavy for their size. The skin should be smooth, without bruises, and deep green in color.
- Beware a zucchini with a hard rind since it is probably past its prime and will have hard seeds and stringy flesh.
- Handle zucchini with care, since it is very fragile, and small punctures will lead to decay.
- Store zucchini in a breathable plastic bag in the refrigerator for up to 1 week. Be sure the zucchini is dry when you put it in the bag because moisture generates mold and spoilage.
- To retain maximum vitamins and fiber, do not peel zucchini.

Be a Fat Flush Cook

- Onion and garlic go well with zucchini, but you can add flavor to zucchini by experimenting with any of the Fat Flush herbs and spices.
- Zucchini's mild flavor blends well with plain yogurt, lemon, olive oil, peppers, mushrooms, or onions.
- Steaming is a great way to prepare zucchini; the finished product is sweet and crisp. You can also grill it, toss it in a stir-fry, or munch on it raw.
- Experiment with zucchini by grating it or cutting it into sticks or rings.
- If you overcook zucchini, you'll end up with mush. If that should happen to you, your best bet is to toss the mushy zucchini in some soup!

THINK TWICE!

- *People who have been diagnosed with kidney or gallbladder problems may want to avoid eating zucchini on a regular basis since it contains oxalates, a substance that can crystallize in the body and cause kidney stones.*
- *If you cut into a zucchini and immediately notice an acrid odor, do not eat it! There have been rare cases in which a compound called*

Cucurbitacin E *has been found in zucchini. It creates extreme bitterness in a zucchini. In addition to the unpleasant smell and bitter flavor, this compound can cause cramps and diarrhea.*

It's Been Said . . .

Who needs potato chips or pretzels? I love to snack on zucchini chips, made by baking thin slices of zucchini in a 350 degree oven for about 15 minutes.

THOMAS D., MARYLAND

CHAPTER

4 Fat Flushing Fruits

Some things you have to do every day. Eating seven apples on Saturday night instead of one a day just isn't going to get the job done.

JIM ROHN

No list of Fat Flushing superfoods would be complete without some colorful, nutrient-rich fruits. Fruits provide a healthy way to satisfy your sweet tooth while filling up on Fat Flushing vitamins, minerals, and fiber.

Because fruits contain a high percentage of water, they help hydrate the body, while, at the same time, their impressive levels of potassium and magnesium work to wring excess water weight from body tissues. Cellulose, the fibrous matter in fruits, provides smooth passage for food in the digestive tract and eases bowel action. This laxative effect is enhanced by the sugar and organic acids in fruit.

Many fruits contain phytochemicals, a group of compounds that helps prevent chronic diseases such as cardiovascular disease, cancer, and diabetes. Fruits are also famous for their antioxidants, which slow down oxidation and prevent cell and tissue damage. Countless studies have shown that eating a variety of fruits helps control blood pressure, prevent heart attacks, strokes, and cancer, and even maintain eye health.

Fruits have what it takes to maintain the body's acid-alkaline balance. In fact, the vitamins, minerals, and enzymes in fruits are extremely beneficial in normalizing all the body's processes. What researchers have discovered is that while fruits contain a number of nutritious elements, it is the *combined* power of all the nutrients working together that gives fruits their disease-fighting abilities. Fat Flushing fruits are a must for a healthy, balanced diet. It's easy to fit them into most any meal—or save them for snack time.

APPLES

Fat Flush Factors

Cholesterol Zapper

Blood-Sugar Stabilizer

Detoxifier

Whether its peel is red, yellow, or green, few things are as refreshing as the crisp, white flesh of an apple. From Adam and Eve to Johnny Appleseed, apples have played an important part in history and mythology. Originally from Eastern Europe and Asia, the apple is one of the oldest cultivated fruits. Certain varieties of apples have been grown for at least 2000 years and, over the centuries, people have developed over 7000 different varieties of apple.

From the crisp, aromatic Braeburn to the green tang of a Granny Smith, apples contain a number of components, namely fiber and flavonoids, that lower cholesterol, improve bowel function, and reduce the risk of heart disease, stroke, cancer, diabetes, and asthma! The research on apples is extensive and varied. The National Cancer Institute reported that flavonoids, a type of antioxidant found in apples, may reduce the risk of lung cancer by up to 50 percent.[1] A group of researchers at the University of California at Davis found that two apples a day may decrease oxidation of LDL cholesterol by up to 34 percent.[2] And, quercitin, a potent flavonoid found in apple peel, has been shown to reduce the risk of heart attack by 32 percent.[3]

Offering both soluble and insoluble fiber, apples are known for aiding digestion and promoting weight loss. Even though they are rich in natural sugar, apples do not cause a rapid rise in blood-sugar levels. The nutritional make up of the apple prevents the body from pumping out too much insulin. In addition, apples contain a natural fibrous chemical called *pectin,* which limits the amount of fat absorbed by your cells. Pectin also grabs toxins, such as the heavy metals lead and mercury, and escorts them out of the body. Studies have shown that because of their pectin, green apples are the best choice for cleansing the liver.

Pectin prevails over the appetite, too. Researchers at Texas's Brooke Army Medical Center studied the impact of pectin on hunger by feeding orange juice to a group of 74 people. Half the people got plain orange juice and half got juice with added pectin. People who received the pectin-laced juice reported having little sense of hunger for 4 hours, while the people who drank regular orange juice complained of hunger much sooner. The researchers concluded that pectin may slow digestion, keeping food in the stomach longer.[4] So, whether you grab an apple as a snack or serve it as a delicious dessert, you'll be cleansing your body and trimming your waistline at the same time.

Recommended Usage: An apple a day.

Just the Facts

- While Washington is famous for its apple orchards, apples are grown in almost every state in the United States.
- The average American eats about 120 apples every year—a far cry from an apple a day!
- Did you ever wonder why it's customary to give an apple to a teacher? This practice began when public school teachers were paid in food or goods, rather than money.
- Researchers at Yale University discovered that some people lowered their blood pressure just by smelling the pleasant scent of spiced apples.[5]

Boost the Benefits

- When you're buying apples, select fruit that is firm, richly colored, and free of soft spots.
- In the northern hemisphere, apple season begins at the end of summer and lasts until early winter. When you buy apples at other times of the year, they have been imported from the southern hemisphere.
- Skip the apple juice and go for the whole apple instead. It provides more nutrition and fiber than the juice.
- To prevent further ripening, store apples in a plastic bag in the refrigerator. They should stay fresh for up to 6 weeks, but it's a good idea to check them regularly and remove any apples that begin to decay before they affect the others.
- Protect apple slices from oxidation and discoloration by dipping them into a solution of one part lemon juice and three parts water.

Be a Fat Flush Cook

- An apple is the perfect portable snack. Experiment with different varieties throughout the year.

- The tarter the apple, the better it maintains its texture during cooking.
- Add diced apples to tossed green salads.
- Simmer a chopped apple in broth with red cabbage.

THINK TWICE!

Commercially raised apples may have been exposed to as many as 10 pesticides. You can avoid consuming these pesticides by removing the skin, but you will be sacrificing both fiber and flavonoids. Your other choices are to purchase organically grown apples or wash your apples in a Clorox bath. (See page 136.)

It's Been Said . . .

I was looking for a Fat Flushing alternative to sweet desserts, so I sliced an apple and shook the slices in a plastic bag with a tablespoon of ground flaxseed and half a teaspoon of cinnamon. Having this treat in the evening has helped me stick to the Fat Flush Plan—and lose 25 pounds!

SANDY M., CALIFORNIA

Comfort me with apples for I am sick.

KING SOLOMON, THE BIBLE

BERRIES

Fat Flush Factors

Detoxifier

Cholesterol Zapper

Energizer

While there are many types of berries—from smooth-skinned varieties to those with fleshy segments—I am focusing on three Fat Flushing favorites: raspberries, strawberries, and blueberries. Raspberries can be traced back to prehistoric times, strawberries have grown wild around the world for thousands of years, and blueberries are native to North America.

Filled with the antioxidant, *ellagic acid,* raspberries help prevent unwanted damage to cell membranes by neutralizing free radicals. Raspberries also contain *flavonoids,* the substances that give them their rich red color. These phytonutrients prevent overgrowth of bacteria and fungi, including Candida albicans—a factor in yeast infections and those pesky carb cravings. Brimming with manganese, vitamin C, a number of B vitamins, and dietary fiber, raspberries benefit the liver by cleansing the blood.

Strawberries reign supreme as the most popular berry in America. They contain the most vitamin C of any berry and plenty of cancer-protective ellagic acid. Phytonutrients called *anthocyanins* give strawberries their inviting red color while packing a potent Fat Flushing punch by breaking down excess toxins in the liver.

As researchers at Tufts University discovered, blueberries provide more antioxidants—including the powerful cholesterol fighter *resveratrol*—than most other common fruits or vegetables.[6] They contain significant amounts of both antibacterial and antiviral compounds, and they may also protect against heart disease and cancer. High in fiber, blueberries also contain *tannins,* which serve to cleanse the digestive system. And they promote a healthy urinary tract by preventing bacterial growth.

All berries are bursting with vitamin C, which stimulates production of carnitine, an amino acid that boosts metabolism. In addition, berries contain natural fructose, which is satisfying to a sweet tooth. Researchers have also found that the insoluble fiber in berries prevents their total calories from being absorbed, making them a tasty Fat Flushing treat![7]

Recommended Usage: Add a handful of berries to your daily diet.

Just the Facts

- Across the United States, fresh blueberries are available for nearly 8 months of the year.
- If all the blueberries grown annually in North America were spread out in a single layer, they would cover a four-lane highway stretching from New York to Chicago.
- Until the 1800s, strawberries remained a luxury food, found only in the kitchens of the wealthy.
- Strawberries are not considered a "true" berry, because they grow from the base of the plant rather than from a flower ovary.
- Currently, the strawberry is the most popular berry in the world, with blueberries coming in a close second.
- If a raspberry's green "cap" is intact, the berry is immature and will never become sweet.

Boost the Benefits

- When you're buying berries, look for plump, firm fruits with a deep, shiny color. Shake the container to see if the berries move freely. If not, the berries may be soft, damaged, or moldy.
- Keep in mind that moisture causes berries to decay. Stay away from berry containers that are stained or wet.
- When purchasing frozen berries, shake the bag gently to check for freely moving berries. If the fruit seems clumped together, the bag may have been thawed and refrozen. Properly handled, frozen berries should keep for about a year.
- Always check berries before storing and remove any damaged berries to prevent the spread of mold.
- Berries may be stored in a covered container in the refrigerator for about 3 to 5 days. However, for optimal health benefits and flavor, plan to serve berries within a day or two after purchasing them.
- Fresh berries—especially raspberries—are very fragile and should be washed briefly and carefully and then gently patted dry. To preserve the texture and flavor of strawberries, wash them *before* you remove their caps.
- You'll notice the fullest flavor if you eat fresh berries at room temperature.

Be a Fat Flush Cook

- Add color and flavor to a mixed green salad by tossing in some sliced strawberries.
- A few ripe raspberries make a beautiful (and delicious) garnish for a salad or dessert.
- Layer sliced strawberries, whole blueberries, and plain yogurt in a wine glass to make a parfait dessert.
- Mix your favorite berry with cinnamon, plain yogurt, and a bit of lemon juice to make a topping for spelt French toast.
- Fresh or frozen berries make a perfect addition to a Fat Flush whey protein smoothie.
- A few luscious frozen strawberries make a refreshing and revitalizing summer snack.

PEACHES

Fat Flush Factors

Detoxifier

Diuretic

Originally from China, peaches have captivated Americans since well before Thomas Jefferson planted 160 peach trees in his orchard. Today, nearly 300 varieties of this succulent fruit thrive in warm climates around the world.

There are two categories of peaches: clingstone and freestone. They are differentiated by how easily the fruit pulls away from the pit. With freestones, the pit comes away easily, but with cling peaches separating the pit is more of a challenge.

Peaches are high in the antioxidant vitamins A and C, which promote beautiful, ageless skin, healthy vision, and a strong immune system. This fuzzy fruit is also a good source of potassium, fiber, and b*eta cryptothanxin*, a phytonutrient recognized for preventing heart disease. And, while peaches are already known to prevent certain types of cancer, new varieties of the fruit are being developed that will yield even higher levels of cancer-fighting antioxidants and phytochemicals.

Peaches have both a diuretic and a laxative effect and help stimulate digestive juices. This nutritious Fat Flushing fruit also contains boron, known to pump up estrogen levels in postmenopausal women, stimulate the brain, and help prevent osteoporosis. So feel free to indulge in a juicy ripe peach whenever you like. It only tastes sinful.

Recommended Usage: Three or four peaches per week.

Just the Facts

- Usually, freestone peaches are sold fresh, while clingstones are canned, frozen, and preserved.
- In ancient China, people believed that the peach conferred immortality on those who ate it. Today, the peach remains a symbol of hope and longevity.
- To pit a peach easily, slice it horizontally all the way around, and then twist the halves apart.

- Because of consumer demand, peaches aren't as fuzzy as they used to be. After being picked, most peaches are mechanically brushed to get rid of some of the fuzz.

Boost the Benefits

- When you're shopping for peaches, go for unblemished fruit that is free of bruises and that has a warm, fragrant aroma.
- Contrary to popular belief, the red blush on peaches is not a measure of ripeness. Instead, look for peaches with a creamy or golden undercolor and pass on peaches with a greenish color. They were picked before they matured and will *never* ripen.
- To test for ripeness, squeeze a peach gently. A peach is prime when it gives to slight pressure and smells sweet.
- If you need to ripen peaches, store them in a loosely closed brown bag at room temperature. Never store fresh peaches in plastic bags. This changes their flavor and texture.
- You can store ripe peaches in the crisper bin of your refrigerator for a few days, but they may lose some of their flavor. Whenever possible, bring them to room temperature before serving.
- Keep in mind that most of a peach's vitamins are in the peel, so eat the whole peach, fuzz and all, whenever possible.

Be a Fat Flush Cook

- Try poaching peaches and serving them as a simple dessert.
- Add peach chunks to a skewer of meat and vegetables for grilling.
- Peaches make a delicious topping for Fat Flush French toast, made with spelt bread.
- Pop some peach slices into a blender with some cranberry juice, whey protein and spices for a satisfying breakfast smoothie.
- Peaches may be baked, grilled, or broiled and served along with your favorite meat or fish dinner.
- For a quick and easy dessert, slice a fresh peach, and then top it with a dollop of plain yogurt and a sprinkling of cinnamon and ground flaxseed.

THINK TWICE!

Peach pits contain a toxic substance known as hydrocyanic acid *or* cyanide *and can be fatal if ingested in large quantities. So be sure to dispose of them properly to keep them away from children and pets.*

CHAPTER

5 Fat Flushing Herbs and Spices

We are indeed much more than what we eat, but what we eat can nevertheless help us to be much more than what we are.

ADELLE DAVIS

For thousands of years, people have utilized herbs and spices to flavor foods and treat illnesses. Sadly, even with the wide array of spices available, black pepper remains the most popular seasoning among Americans!

I invite you to expand your use of herbs and spices to include a variety of Fat Flushing flavors. For example, seasoning your foods with a bit of cayenne, coriander, or cumin goes a long way toward boosting the nutritional value of your meal and helps you steer clear of bloat-promoting salt and artificial additives.

What's the difference between an herb and a spice? An herb is an aromatic leaf, like parsley, while a spice stems from a pungent seed, root, or bark, such as cinnamon. Both types of seasonings offer a myriad of Fat Flushing benefits, from urging the metabolism into high gear, to erasing excess water weight.

Antioxidants, so abundant in herbs and spices, have become synonymous with good health because of their ability to neutralize harmful free radicals in the body. In addition, these Fat Flushing seasonings aid the digestive process, support the liver, and help prevent disease. To achieve the greatest impact from seasonings, make use of the full range of Fat Flushing herbs and spices. Avoid using any of the seasonings every day to prevent the development of food allergies. (People are prone to develop allergies to foods they eat all the time.)

The facts are indisputable. Herbs and spices transform the simplest meal by providing flavor and soul to your food. At the same time, they impart a host of nutritional rewards. What more could you ask for from a *sprinkle of this* and a *dash of that*?

ANISE

Fat Flush Factor

Diuretic

What smells like licorice, tastes like licorice, but isn't licorice? It's anise, one of the oldest cultivated spices in the world. Native to the Middle East, anise has been used as a medicine since prehistoric times. Romans used anise to thwart indigestion, prevent bad dreams, treat scorpion bites, and ward off the evil eye. In the sixteenth century, anise served as bait in mousetraps. These days, we have tastier uses for anise. It flavors cakes, cookies, and breads; and enriches soups, stews, and seafood. From liqueurs to licorice candy, anise lends its distinctive flavor to a wide variety of food and drink.

Beyond the kitchen, anise is found in many commercial cough syrups and sore throat medications. In addition to adding flavor to these drugs, anise contains the chemicals *creosol* and *alpha-pinene,* which have been shown to loosen mucus in the bronchial tubes, thus making it easier to cough up. Studies have confirmed that *anethole,* the main active ingredient in anise, inhibits the growth of certain tumors, especially colon cancer. And scientists at the University of California found that anethole helps fight Candida albicans—those sugar-loving yeast microbes that can wreak havoc in our bodies.[1]

Consuming anise can soothe a queasy stomach, boost antioxidant levels, and, because it contains *dianethole* and *photoanethole,* which are chemically similar to estrogen, can even take the edge off perimenopausal symptoms.

Recommended Usage: Up to 1 teaspoon of anise seeds per week.

Just the Facts

- Licorice candy contains very little "licorice." Instead, most of its flavor comes from anise.
- Mexico is the world's largest producer of anise.
- Anise "perfumes" the artificial rabbit used in greyhound races.
- In medicine, anise oil masks the taste of bitter-tasting drugs.

Be a Fat Flush Cook

- For refreshing taste, sprinkle a few anise seeds onto a salad, or mix some into your salad dressing.
- When you're cooking cabbage, add anise seeds to produce a delightful flavor.
- Sprinkle a bit of ground anise in hot lemon water. Drink it first thing in the morning to give your digestive system a boost.
- Baked apples are delicious with ground anise seed sprinkled on top.
- Store anise in a cool, dry, dark place in tightly sealed containers. Anise may retain its flavor qualities and strength for up to 3 years.

It's Been Said . . .

Once you get a spice in your home, you have it forever. Women never throw out spices. The Egyptians were buried with their spices. I know which one I'm taking with me when I go.

ERMA BOMBECK

Try steeping a teaspoon of anise seeds in hot water to make a Fat Flush-friendly tea. It makes a refreshing and elegant drink after dinner.

CINDY C., CALIFORNIA

CAYENNE

Fat Flush Factors

Thermogenic

Energizer

Cayenne has been used as both food and medicine in the tropical areas of South and Central America and Africa for more than 7000 years. Related to both mild bell peppers and fiery chili peppers, cayenne bears no connection to black pepper. In fact, it was Spanish explorers who misnamed cayenne a pepper and began trading it around the world.

Cayenne does much more than create a tongue-tingling meal. It is loaded with vitamins C, B, and A and also contains calcium, phosphorus, and iron. One of the richest sources of vitamin E, cayenne helps keep the heart healthy and strong. And, as its bright red color suggests, it provides us with immune-boosting beta-carotene, one of the most important antioxidants in the body. Cayenne offers additional value as a painkiller (especially against the discomfort of arthritis), an antiseptic, and a digestive aid.

As most of us can attest, cayenne is a diaphoretic—a sweat-inducing spice. Its hotness comes from a high concentration of *capsicum,* a substance that has been firing up the circulation for centuries. It is capsicum that gives cayenne the power to get the blood pumping efficiently, stimulate the body's metabolic rate, and help clean fat out of the arteries.

A study at Oxford Polytechnic Institute proved that cayenne pepper stimulates the metabolism by about 20 percent and results in increased distribution of oxygen throughout the body.[2]

Recommended Usage: Liberal use, to taste, every other day.

Just the Facts

- Capsicum, the colorless, heat-producing compound in cayenne, is also known as *capsaicin*. Amazingly, within the last few years, over 1300 studies on capsicum have been published in medical journals.
- Because of its hot, burning flavor, cayenne takes its name from a Greek word meaning "to bite."

- People who break out in a sweat after eating cayenne are experiencing "gustatory perspiration."
- Dropping a pinch of cayenne into your gloves will keep your hands warm on a cold morning.

Boost the Benefits

- You may see cayenne ranging in color from deep red to nearly orange.
- Cayenne is one of the few spices that is always purchased in ground form.
- Cayenne pepper should be kept in a tightly sealed glass jar, away from direct sunlight. Stored in this way, it should keep up to 1 year.

Be a Fat Flush Cook

- Cayenne is sure to heat up any combination of mixed, steamed veggies.
- Give your herbal coffee a traditional Mexican flair by adding a tiny bit of cayenne pepper.
- Adding cayenne and lemon juice to cooked bitter greens, such as kale, really complements the flavor.
- Use cayenne in moderation. For example, for a recipe that serves four, start with just a dash or two. Increase the amount, dash by dash, until you have the heat level you desire.
- Because cayenne's heat intensifies when it's frozen, you may want to go easy when making a dish destined for the freezer.

THINK TWICE!

- *Keep cayenne away from your eyes and moist mucous membranes.*
- *When making smoothies, don't mistake your bottle of cayenne for cinnamon. This happened to one unlucky Fat Flusher who experienced a whole new taste sensation that morning!*

It's Been Said . . .

I've banished my salt and pepper shakers. Instead, I keep a container of cayenne on the table so I can rev up my metabolism at most every meal.

JULIE T., WASHINGTON

CINNAMON

Fat Flush Factors

Thermogenic

Blood-Sugar Stabilizer

Once considered a precious commodity, cinnamon boasts a long history as both a spice and a medicine. Cinnamon is actually tree bark and can be found in dried stick form or as a ground powder. "True" cinnamon comes from Ceylon and is difficult to find in U.S. stores. Tan in color, it offers a delicate aroma and a sweeter flavor than the more common, less expensive "cassia" cinnamon. If the cinnamon in your cupboard is mahogany red, it is cassia and was probably grown in Vietnam, China, Indonesia, or Central America.

Medieval physicians treated coughs, sore throats, and diarrhea with cinnamon. Europeans used cinnamon to preserve foods and to mask the stench and flavor of spoiling meats. And it turns out that they were on to something. Recent studies have confirmed cinnamon's ability to rid foods of dangerous bacteria. One study, conducted at Kansas State University, found that cinnamon destroyed E. coli bacteria in apple juice.[3]

The healing powers of cinnamon's active ingredients (*cinnamaldehyde, cinnamyl acetate*, and *cinnamyl alcohol*) don't end there. Cinnamon has been well researched for its ability to prevent unwanted clumping of blood platelets. Cinnamon consumption can boost the metabolism and derail Candida, the microorganism that causes yeast overgrowth in the body. The calcium and fiber content of cinnamon seems to improve intestinal health and protect against heart disease. And, best of all, in both test-tube and animal studies, scientists at the U.S. Department of Agriculture have found that cinnamon makes cells more responsive to insulin.[4] Clinical trials with humans are currently underway, but it appears that just a dash of cinnamon can help the body to metabolize glucose, keeping blood-sugar levels in check.

Recommended Usage: 1/2 to 1 teaspoon, every other day.

Just the Facts

- In the United States, consumption of cinnamon has jumped by 6.5 million pounds in the last decade.
- Most of the "cinnamon" sold across the United States is actually cassia (although it is labeled as cinnamon). Cinnamon and cassia are

closely related, but cassia is stronger and less delicate in flavor. True cinnamon is readily available in other countries, including Mexico.

- Cinnamon sticks are known officially as "quills."
- If you consume cinnamon every day, your body may stop responding to its thermogenic properties.

Boost the Benefits

- How can you tell if your cinnamon sticks are true cinnamon or cassia? True cinnamon quills curl up from one side, like a jellyroll, while cassia quills roll inward from both sides, like a scroll.
- To ensure the best flavor and nutrition from your cinnamon, buy it in small quantities because it becomes stale quickly, losing both flavor and aroma. Your best bet is to grind your own cinnamon from quills, using a spice or coffee grinder.
- Keep your cinnamon in a tightly sealed, glass container in a cool, dark, and dry place. Ground cinnamon keeps for about 6 months, while cinnamon sticks stay fresh for about 1 year. To check for freshness, *smell* your cinnamon. Discard it if the aroma is no longer sweet.
- Foods that undergo radiation during their processing may form free radicals that are potentially harmful to humans. Look for organically grown cinnamon, because it has likely not been irradiated. Among other potentially harmful effects, irradiating cinnamon can reduce its vitamin C and carotenoid content.

Be a Fat Flush Cook

- To prevent the bitterness that comes with extended cooking, add ground cinnamon to your dish shortly before you serve it.
- Try a dash of cinnamon in spaghetti sauce, beef stew, or chili.
- Brighten the flavor of apple, peach, or pear slices with a sprinkle of cinnamon.
- Before broiling, season chicken breasts or lamb chops with some sweet-spicy cinnamon.
- Give a healthy twist to cinnamon toast by drizzling flaxseed oil onto spelt toast and then sprinkling it with cinnamon.

Fat Flushing Fun

To fill your home with the scent of cinnamon, simmer a quill or two in a pot of water. This is especially nice throughout the winter holidays.

It's Been Said . . .

To give your stir-fry a Middle Eastern flair, simmer a cinnamon quill in a few tablespoons of broth until it unrolls, then add your other ingredients.

PATTY R., TEXAS

CLOVES

Fat Flush Factor

Thermogenic

Did you know that cloves are actually flower buds, picked and dried before they blossomed? Shaped like nails, whole cloves are an easy spice to recognize and have been prized throughout the ages. In ancient China, people were required to freshen their mouths by chewing cloves prior to meeting the emperor, and, in the Spice Islands, wars were fought over the right to grow and sell cloves. Today, Brazil, Indonesia, and Zanzibar all produce cloves, although the finest cloves are said to come from Madagascar.

Eugenol, the main component of cloves, has a long-standing reputation for killing bacteria and viruses. This explains why cloves have been valued throughout history as a food preservative, a wound disinfectant, and a toothache cure. Highly antiseptic, clove oil continues to be used in mouthwashes, medicines, and antacids today.

As a Fat Flushing food, cloves stimulate digestion, fire up the metabolism, and reduce intestinal bloating and gas. So keep this hot, slightly sweet spice handy. You can try whole cloves to give an intense "punch" to your food, or use ground cloves for a more subdued flavor.

Recommended Usage: 1/8 to 1/4 teaspoon, two to three times per week.

Just the Facts

- Cloves serve as natural insect repellents for ants and other crawling insects.
- Cloves are the only spice that is smoked more than it is eaten. Indonesia uses half the world's supply of cloves to make "kretek" cigarettes. (The American Lung Association has declared that clove cigarettes are even more toxic than tobacco.[5])

Boost the Benefits

- Because of their high oil content, you need to keep cloves tightly covered or they will lose flavor and turn rancid. Store this spice away from the light, in an airtight container.

- Look for whole cloves that are mahogany red, are slightly oily, and give off a pungent, sweet aroma. Avoid black or shriveled cloves; they are not fresh.
- Get rid of any ground clove that tastes bitter or harsh. It's too old.

Be a Fat Flush Cook

- Use cloves sparingly because the flavor continues to develop in a dish over time.
- Add cloves to tomato dishes or sprinkle them over cooked sweet potato.
- Do you make your own broth? Push a clove or two into an onion to give a distinctive flavor to chicken or vegetable broth.

It's Been Said . . .

Several times a week, I add a pinch of cloves to my morning smoothie. It's especially good in a peach smoothie!

CAROL A., CALIFORNIA

CORIANDER

Fat Flush Factor

Blood-Sugar Stabilizer

Coriander. Is it an herb or a spice? How about *both*? The fresh minty-sweet leaves are considered an herb and are sometimes called cilantro or Chinese parsley. The seeds, which look like tan peppercorns, are a fragrant spice and taste like a mixture of sweet orange peel and sage.

Coriander is probably one of the first herbs to be used by people, going back as far as 5000 B.C. If you read *Tales of the Arabian Nights*, you'll see coriander mentioned as an aphrodisiac. In ancient China, eating coriander was a way to ensure immortality. Coriander holds the honor of being one of the first spices to arrive in America, and it sits high on the list of the healing spices.

Coriander is traditionally known as an "antidiabetic" plant. This claim has recently been confirmed. The *British Journal of Nutrition* published a study which found that when coriander was added to the diet of diabetic mice, it helped stimulate their secretion of insulin and lowered their blood sugar.[6]

Currently, scientists are taking a look at coriander for its cholesterol-lowering effects. Researchers at a university in India fed coriander to rats that were on a high-fat, high-cholesterol diet. They found that coriander lowered levels of total and LDL cholesterol while actually increasing HDL levels.[7, 8] While further research is needed, there is no doubt that coriander packs a wallop as a Fat Flushing food.

Recommended Usage: Up to one bunch per week.

Just the facts

- Coriander stalks are tender and have the same flavor as the leaves—so don't throw them out!
- Only a small amount of coriander is needed to flavor dishes, especially if you're using fresh coriander.

Boost the Benefits

- When buying fresh coriander, look for vibrantly deep green leaves that are firm, crisp, and unspotted.

- Fresh coriander leaves are perishable and won't keep more than a few days. To maximize storage time, wrap the leaves in a moist cloth and refrigerate them in a loosely fitting plastic bag. If the roots are intact, store the bouquet of coriander in a glass of water and cover it loosely with a plastic bag.
- Bunched coriander can be frozen by simply wrapping it in foil before placing it in the freezer.
- To keep coriander seeds, either whole or ground, store them in a tightly sealed container away from light. Ground coriander keeps for about 4 months, while whole seeds stay fresh for at least 1 year.
- Wash and chop fresh coriander right before adding it to your dish since the aroma of coriander intensifies immediately after being cut. To clean your coriander, place it in a bowl of cold water and swish it around with your hands. Repeat this process with clean water until no dirt remains in the bowl.
- To intensify the flavor of whole coriander seeds, toast them in a dry, nonstick frying pan before you grind them.

Be a Fat Flush Cook

- To enjoy the peak flavor of fresh coriander leaves, add them to your dish during the last few moments of cooking.
- Season fish with lemon juice, coriander, and mustard. Then broil for delectable flavor.
- Stir-fry some spinach, fresh garlic, and coriander seeds. Season with ginger and cumin and you've got a side dish that's jam packed with nutrients.
- Substitute fresh coriander for parsley or chervil in most any recipe.
- Toss fresh coriander leaves with salad greens for an added zing.

It's Been Said . . .

I put coriander seeds in a pepper mill and keep it on the dinner table to give many of my Fat Flush meals an extra boost of flavor.

CARYL P., NORTH CAROLINA

CUMIN

Fat Flush Factor

Detoxifier

An ordinary-looking seed, cumin packs a punch when it comes to both flavor and health benefits. Cumin has a distinctive taste, slightly bitter and peppery with a hint of citrus, which it lends to a wide array of Mexican, Indian, and Middle Eastern dishes. In the kitchens of ancient Greece and Rome, cumin served as a replacement for black pepper, which was expensive and hard to come by. During the Middle Ages, Europeans recognized cumin as a symbol of love and fidelity. Wives baked loaves of cumin bread to give to their husbands as they headed off to war.

Today, cumin is experiencing a comeback, as more people come to appreciate its culinary and therapeutic properties. Cumin seed is high in protein, potassium, iron, and thiamine. Researchers are finding that cumin stimulates the secretion of pancreatic enzymes, thereby aiding digestion and absorption of nutrients. Because of its ability to scavenge for free radicals, cumin enhances the detoxification process in the liver. And, two of cumin's active ingredients, *carevol* and *limonene*, have been shown to be powerful cancer fighters.

Whether you select the black or yellow-brown variety, be sure to add a healthy dose of cumin to your diet. Your liver will thank you.

Recommended Usage: Liberal use, to taste, every other day.

Just the Facts

- Cumin ranks as one of the most popular spices in the world, second only to black pepper.
- Cumin "seeds" are actually the small dried fruits of the cumin plant.
- Cumin is the essential ingredient in chili powder.

Boost the Benefits

- Whether whole or ground, cumin seeds should be stored in tightly sealed glass containers in a cool, dry place. Ground cumin keeps for about 6 months, while the whole seeds stay fresh for up to 1 year.

- Whenever possible, buy whole cumin seeds instead of powder since ground cumin loses its flavor more quickly than the seeds. You can easily grind your own cumin with a mortar and pestle.
- To bring out their full aroma and flavor, lightly roast whole cumin seeds before using them in a recipe.
- When making a dish that needs to simmer for a long time, consider using *whole* cumin seeds. Ground cumin can quickly lose its strength and become bitter.

Be a Fat Flush Cook

- Add cumin to beef to give a new twist to pot roast or stew recipes.
- Flavor lamb brochettes or kabobs with cumin, and then grill.
- Season steamed vegetables with cumin to give them a North African flair.

It's Been Said . . .

On those days when I'm not planning a meal with cumin, I make myself a cup of warming cumin tea by boiling the seeds in water and then letting them steep for 8 to10 minutes.

DONNA F., PENNSYLVANIA

DILL

Fat Flush Factor

Diuretic

Dill offers double the pleasure—and Fat Flushing power—since *both* its leaves and seeds may be used as a seasoning. Dill's fernlike, green leaves are delicate and have a soft, sweet taste. Dried dill seeds are light brown ovals, with a sweet, citrusy flavor.

One of the favorite herbs in ancient Greece and Rome, dill was considered good luck and was often placed in a baby's cradle or over a door jamb for protection. Ancient soldiers applied roasted dill seeds to their wounds to encourage healing and help prevent infection. Today, we know those soldiers were on to something. Current research has confirmed that dill prevents bacterial overgrowth.[9]

In addition to serving as a natural diuretic, dill weed contains a substance called *carvone*, which aids and calms digestion by relieving intestinal gas. This probably explains why, in early America, children were given dill seeds to calm them during lengthy church services. It also explains why I promote the frequent use of dill. The digestive tract works less efficiently as we age, and consuming dill gives it a welcomed boost.

As an added bonus, the active ingredients in dill qualify it as a "chemoprotective" food that helps neutralize certain carcinogens, such as the *benzopyrenes* found in cigarette smoke, charcoal grill smoke, and the smoke produced by trash incinerators. So use dill liberally to detox your body and delight your taste buds.

Recommended Usage: Two teaspoons per week.

Just the Facts

- It takes a tablespoon of chopped fresh dill to equal one teaspoon of dried dill weed.
- An ounce of dill seeds contains more than 10,000 tiny seeds.
- One tablespoon of dill seed contains as much calcium as a cup of milk. Dill is also a good source of fiber, iron, and magnesium.

Boost the Benefits

- When shopping for fresh dill, look for feathery green leaves. Don't worry if the leaves appear slightly wilted because they usually droop very quickly after being picked.
- Store fresh dill in the refrigerator either wrapped in a damp paper towel or with its stems placed in a container of water—like a bouquet of flowers. Since it is very fragile, dill keeps fresh for only a few days, even if stored properly.
- Forget using a knife and cutting board. Snip fresh dill with scissors to mince the delicate leaves.
- Your best bet for long-term storage is to freeze dill leaves. To use the frozen leaves, just snip off what you need and drop the rest back in the freezer. (Dill tends to darken a bit in the freezer, but it keeps nicely for several months.)
- For handy access when making soups, stews or stir-fries, freeze dill leaves in ice-cube trays covered with broth. Then pop out just as many cubes as you need.
- Keep dried dill seeds in a tightly sealed, glass container. If you keep the container in a cool, dry, dark place, the dill seeds will stay fresh for about 6 months.
- There is no comparison between the flavor of fresh dill and dried dill weed. Use fresh for the most intense flavor. If you must use dried, do so with a generous hand.

Fat Flush Fun

Rumor has it that if you sprinkle some fresh dill leaves in your bath water, you will be irresistible to your lover!

Be a Fat Flush Cook

- The longer dill weed is cooked, the more the flavor diminishes. Add it at the last minute to achieve full flavor and aroma.
- Combine dill weed with plain yogurt and chopped cucumber for a delicious cooling dip or tangy seafood sauce.
- When broiling lamb chops or steak, sprinkle chopped fresh dill on the meat during the last 5 minutes.
- Is fish on the menu? The flavor of dill enhances most fish very well, especially salmon and trout.
- Since dill seeds are known for soothing the stomach after a meal, put some seeds in a small dish and pass it around the dinner table for everyone to enjoy.

DRIED MUSTARD

Fat Flush Factor

Thermogenic

Can you guess what mustard and broccoli have in common? They are both members of the cruciferous family of vegetables. While there are about 40 different types of mustard plants, we get seeds from three main varieties: black, white, and brown mustard. For the most pungent flavor, look for *black* mustard seeds. *White* mustard seeds are the mildest and are used to make American yellow mustard. Dijon mustard contains the flavorful, dark yellow seeds of the *brown* mustard plant.

At first, mustard was considered a medicine rather than a food. In the sixth century B.C., Greek scientist Pythagoras used mustard to take the bite out of scorpion stings. One hundred years later, Hippocrates treated patients with mustard medicines and poultices. Around the globe, people in every culture continued to find uses for mustard. German folklore encouraged brides who wanted to rule the roost to sew mustard seeds into the hem of their wedding dresses, while from Denmark to India mustard was sprinkled around the outside of homes to ward off evil spirits. It was the early Romans who ground mustard seeds and mixed them with wine into a paste similar to the prepared mustards of today.

Mustard seeds contain ample amounts of phytonutrients, including *isothiocyanates.* The isothiocyanates in mustard seeds have been the focus of many cancer-related studies and have been shown to inhibit the growth of existing cancer cells, especially in gastrointestinal tumors.

Mustard seeds provides selenium, magnesium, monounsaturated fats, and phosphorous. And they are a good source of iron, calcium, zinc, and manganese. Best of all, mustard helps flush fat by revving your metabolism. In a study conducted at the Oxford Polytechnic Institute in England, scientists found that spicy foods, especially mustard, spiked metabolic rates by 25 percent.[10] By adding mustard to a meal, participants burned off at least 45 extra calories during the next 3 hours. So skip sugar-filled ketchup and stock up on dried mustard instead. Your waistline will thank you.

Recommended Usage: Liberal use, to taste, every other day.

Just the Facts

- Dry mustard contains at least twice the flavor zip of prepared mustard.
- The Fat Flushing spice, tumeric, is what gives most American mustards their bright yellow color.
- In the United States, pepper is the only spice consumed more often than mustard. And, around the world, people eat over 700 million pounds of mustard every year.
- One teaspoon of dried mustard equals one tablespoon of prepared mustard.

Boost the Benefits

- When you mix dried mustard powder with cold water, a chemical reaction occurs between two enzymes which enhances the pungency and heat of the mustard. To stop the enzymatic process—and turn *down* the heat—you can add some very hot water or a bit of apple cider vinegar. Or just give it time. The mixture will reach its peak in fire and flavor after about 15 minutes and will quickly decline from that point on.
- Store whole mustard seeds in airtight containers in a cool, dry place for up to 1 year. Ground and powdered mustard stays fresh for up to 6 months.

Fat Flushing Fun

- Try this tip during cold weather: Sprinkle dry mustard inside your shoes to prevent cold feet and frostbite.
- Color your world yellow. Use mustard powder as a fertilizer—you'll get brighter-colored daffodils.

Be a Fat Flush Cook

- You may purchase mustard seeds either whole (and grind them yourself) or as a ground powder.
- For a tangy Fat Flushing meal, dredge chicken breasts in "homemade" mustard and bake. Or, use your mustard mixture as a dip for grilled chicken breast, fruits, and vegetables.
- Be creative with ground mustard, but go easy and taste along the way. You can always add more mustard, but there is no "cure" for overdoing it.

THINK TWICE!!

- *Mustard seeds contain goitrogens, naturally occurring substances that can interfere with the functioning of the thyroid gland. If you have been diagnosed with a thyroid disorder, you may want to avoid ground mustard seeds.*
- *Easy does it when you're making your own mustard. Depending on the mustard powder, it's possible to make a mixture that actually burns or blisters your skin.*
- *Mustard contains sulfur, so steer clear if you have an allergy to sulfur.*

It's Been Said . . .

My family loves Ann Louise's basic fat flushing salad dressing as much as I do. Just mix equal parts flax oil and apple cider vinegar. Add dried mustard, fresh garlic, and minced dill to taste.

CANDY C., KENTUCKY

Mustard's no good without roast beef.

CHICO MARX, MONKEY BUSINESS

FENNEL SEED

Fat Flush Factor

Diuretic

Looking like tiny watermelons, greenish-gray fennel seeds give foods a subtle, sweet, licoricelike flavor. Yet fennel's reputation through the ages has been as a digestive soother. These unassuming little seeds can calm an acidic stomach, ease irritable bowel syndrome, and alleviate gas pains. As an added bonus, fennel relieves bloating by acting as a natural diuretic. How can this herb, which the Chinese used as a remedy for snake bites and scorpion stings, have such a soothing effect on the body? It appears that fennel relaxes smooth muscles in the body, including the lining of the digestive and urinary tracts.

Recent research suggests that *anethole,* the active ingredient in fennel, has an estrogenlike activity, making it a potential remedy for the symptoms of perimenopause. Anethole may also support the liver by encouraging regeneration of liver cells, although more research is necessary to confirm this.[11]

So whether you reach for fennel to season your food or chew a few seeds to settle your stomach after a big meal, you'll reap the benefits of this aromatic herb.

Recommended Usage: A maximum of 1 teaspoon of fennel seeds every other day. (The stems and the fronds may be eaten freely.)

Just the Facts

- Fennel comes from the Greek word for "marathon" because an ancient battle between the Greeks and the Persians was fought at Marathon on a field of fennel.
- "Bulb fennel" is a *vegetable* that resembles a plump celery plant.

Boost the Benefits

- To purchase good-quality fennel, look for seeds that are either yellow or greenish-brown and that taste and smell a bit like licorice.
- Toasting fennel seeds enhances their flavor.

Be a Fat Flush Cook

- Typically used to complement fish, fennel is also found in a variety of Italian dishes.
- Sprinkle fennel and garlic on broiled lamb chops for a fabulous flavor.
- Add fennel to your favorite meatloaf recipe, sprinkle it over an apple before baking, or use a few seeds to season your next omelet.
- Fennel and fish are made for each other. Try adding some fennel seeds to the basting juices during cooking.

THINK TWICE!

- *If you have a history of an estrogen-dependant cancer, avoid fennel in significant quantities until more research is completed on fennel's estrogenic activity.*
- *Because it closely resembles poison hemlock, don't pick fennel in the wild unless you are an experienced herb harvester. Instead, rely on the fennel found at your local grocery.*

It's Been Said . . .

To make one slender, take fennel, seeth it in water and drink it first and last, and it shall swaze either him or her.

THE GOOD HOUSEWIFE'S JEWELL, *1585*

For a terrific Fat Flushing entrée, season a salmon steak with fennel, lemon juice and a hint of garlic. Bake or broil and enjoy!"

MAUREEN D., MARYLAND

GARLIC

Fat Flush Factors

Energizer

Detoxifier

What would you expect to pay for a substance that can fight cancer, AIDS, and heart disease, lower both cholesterol and blood pressure by 10 percent, and serve as a natural antibiotic and antifungal medication? Put your calculators away. Garlic does all this and much more—for about 15 cents per clove. Mother Nature gave us the gift of garlic—a Fat Flushing food that has been utilized as both food and medicine for over 5000 years.

The health benefits of garlic are noted in both the Bible and the Talmud, and an Egyptian papyrus from 1500 B.C. recommends garlic as a treatment for a variety of ailments—from dog bites to bladder infections. Today, garlic is being heavily researched, and we have learned that it serves as a diuretic, a stimulant, and a sweat promoter. It stimulates the metabolism, stabilizes blood-sugar levels, and eliminates toxins from the body.

Garlic contains a wide range of trace minerals, including copper, iron, zinc, magnesium, germanium, and especially selenium. In addition, garlic contains sulfur compounds, vitamins A and C, fiber, and various amino acids. In all, garlic provides more than 100 biologically useful chemicals. The "active" component of garlic is a sulfur compound known as *allicin*. This compound is generated only when a garlic clove is broken, and it is what gives raw, cut garlic its distinctive odor and pungent taste. Allicin also gives garlic its powerful Fat Flushing punch. At least 12 studies have confirmed that allicin clears cholesterol from the blood. The largest study, conducted by German researchers on 261 participants, reported that total cholesterol levels dropped by 12 percent in 12 weeks in the group treated with garlic.[12]

Recommended Usage: Two to six garlic cloves every other day.

Just the Facts

- One clove of garlic that's been pushed through a garlic press is ten times stronger than one clove minced fine with a sharp knife.

- Chewing caraway seeds, fennel seeds, or fresh parsley after eating garlic helps freshen your breath.
- If you plant an individual garlic clove, it will reproduce an entire bulb in about 9 months.

Boost the Benefits

- When you're shopping for garlic, look for plump, firm bulbs with plenty of dry, unbroken skin. Heads that show signs of sprouting are past their prime and were probably not dried properly. Garlic that is very old will crumble when it is gently squeezed.
- Store your garlic in a cool, dark, well-ventilated area, away from potatoes and onions. Do not refrigerate or keep in plastic containers. If stored in a damp, warm environment, garlic will sprout or become moldy.
- Unbroken garlic bulbs will keep for up to 3 months. Individual cloves stay fresh for about 1 week.
- To ensure proper digestion of garlic, make sure you remove the green "germ" in the middle of the clove.

Fat Flushing Fun

Don't try this at home! A famous French chef claims his success comes from chewing a small clove of garlic and then breathing gently on the salad before serving it.

Be a Fat Flush Cook

- To loosen garlic skin, place a clove on a cutting board and cover it with the flat side of a wide knife. Rap the blade sharply with your fist. Don't apply too much pressure because the clove can easily be smashed.
- With garlic, the finer the chop, the stronger the taste. To lightly "perfume" your food with a mild garlic flavor, use whole, unbroken garlic cloves. Thin slices will provide more than a hint of garlic. For a fuller flavor, mince the garlic. And, for in-your-face garlic taste, crush the cloves to a pulp.

THINK TWICE!

- *People who have bleeding disorders or who take anticoagulant medication should consult a doctor before using a garlic supplement or consuming large amounts of garlic.*

- *Stored at room temperature, garlic-in-oil mixtures provide perfect conditions for producing botulism toxin (low acidity, no free oxygen in the oil, and warm temperatures). Do not store raw or roasted garlic in oil at room temperature. You may store the mixture in the refrigerator for up to 1 week.*

It's Been Said . . .

A nickel will get you on the subway, but garlic will get you a seat.

OLD NEW YORK YIDDISH SAYING

I like to rub some crushed garlic on the inside of my salad bowl before adding the salad ingredients. And, making garlic toast is easy with spelt bread, flax oil, and minced garlic!

MICHELLE F., INDIANA

GINGER

Fat Flush Factors

Energizer

Detoxifier

More than 5000 years ago, the ancient Chinese and Indians regarded ginger as a "universal medicine." Today, ginger can be found in more than half of traditional herbal remedies. Throughout its long history, ginger has been used as a remedy for at least 40 conditions, as diverse as diarrhea, dizziness, menstrual cramps, and mumps.

Highly concentrated with active substances, including powerful antioxidants called "gingerols," ginger boasts a number of Fat Flushing benefits. It revs circulation and promotes healthy sweating, encouraging detoxification of the body. Ginger supports liver function, clears up clogged arteries and lowers serum cholesterol levels by nearly 30 percent.[13] It contains compounds that resemble our digestive enzymes, assisting us to digest protein-rich meals more easily. And, according to an Australian study published in the *Journal of Obesity*, ginger raises body temperature and assists the body to burn 20 percent more calories.[14]

While hardly glamorous looking, with its knobby, gnarled appearance, ginger is a versatile and delicious Fat Flushing food. The underground ginger stem, or *rhizome*, is a clump of flattish handlike shapes ranging in color from pale greenish yellow to ivory. The aroma is pungent, and the flavor is peppery and slightly sweet.

Recommended Usage: At least 1/4 inch slice of fresh ginger, every other day.

Just the Facts

- Ginger grows in many tropical areas including southern China, Japan, West Africa, and the Caribbean islands. Jamaican ginger is considered to be the best of all.
- Ginger is generally available in two forms, either young or mature. Most supermarkets carry mature ginger, which has a tough skin that must be peeled. Young ginger, usually found only in Asian markets, does not require peeling.

- Ginger is a good source of calcium, phosphorus, iron, potassium, and Vitamin A.
- Powdered ginger mixed with a bit of sea salt makes an excellent toothpaste, helping to strengthen gums and prevent bad breath.

Boost the Benefits

- Look for firm, plump "fingers" of fresh ginger, with clean, smooth skin. The smaller fingers tend to have the strongest flavor.
- When ginger is fresh, the flesh is pale yellow and very juicy. As it ages, it dries out and becomes fibrous, so avoid ginger that has become discolored, wrinkled, or moldy.
- The new little sprouts that appear on the sides of a ginger root offer a delicate flavor, so don't be afraid to use them.
- Whenever possible, choose fresh ginger over dried because fresh ginger tastes better *and* provides higher levels of gingerol.
- Fresh ginger can be stored in the refrigerator for up to 3 weeks if it is left unpeeled. Stored unpeeled in the freezer, it will keep for up to 6 months.
- Keep dried ginger powder in a tightly sealed, glass container in a cool, dark, and dry place. Better yet, store it in the refrigerator to extend its shelf life to at least 1 year.

Be a Fat Flush Cook

- To substitute fresh ginger for ground ginger in your recipes, use a 1-inch piece of freshly grated ginger root for every 1/4 teaspoon of ground ginger.
- To peel ginger, use the edge of a spoon to scrape the skin off. It should almost roll off—without wasting any of the flesh.
- Spice up cranberry juice with some freshly grated ginger.
- Grate some fresh ginger onto your Fat Flushing sweet potatoes.
- To create a flavor base for a stir-fry, mince some fresh ginger and sauté it in broth with some garlic.
- Add grated ginger and ground flaxseed to apples and bake for a yummy dessert.
- Give zip to a rainbow of sautéed vegetables by adding freshly minced ginger.

THINK TWICE!

Did you know that ginger is a blood thinner? So, if you are taking a prescription blood thinner, avoid ingesting ginger.

It's Been Said . . .

Don't be afraid to spice up that a.m. smoothie. A big chunk of fresh ginger (about a square inch) will give it a bit of zing and help your metabolism.

MARY D., FLORIDA

An I had but one penny in the world, thou should'st have it to buy ginger-bread.

WILLIAM SHAKESPEARE

PARSLEY

Fat Flush Factor

Diuretic

Parsley is the most widely used herb in the United States, yet every year, tons of this green garnish ends up in the garbage. You should think twice about ignoring those decorative sprigs because parsley contains more beta-carotene than carrots, more vitamin C than oranges, more calcium than a cup of milk, and twice as much iron as spinach. It is also a good source of niacin, vitamin B^6, folate, phosphorus, zinc, copper, and fiber.

Through the ages, parsley has been used as a blood purifier and a natural diuretic. Its ability to rid the body of excess water and toxins makes it a shoo-in as a Fat Flushing food. Parsley's high nutritional value gives it the power to promote good digestion, nourish the liver, and strengthen the adrenal glands. In addition, parsley contains the essential oil, *apiole,* which helps stimulate the kidneys and fight water retention. By making parsley part of your regular diet, you can lower your heart rate, reduce your blood pressure, and banish monthly bloat. As an added benefit, the high chlorophyll content in parsley will keep your breath fresh and sweet.

Recommended Usage: One bunch of fresh parsley per week.

Just the Facts

- The Greeks crowned the victors of ancient games with parsley wreaths.
- In the Hebrew celebration of Passover, parsley symbolizes spring and rebirth.
- While there are more than 30 varieties of parsley, curly-leaf parsley, a common garnish, is the most popular, and Italian, or flat-leaf parsley, offers the best flavor for cooking.
- It takes 12 pounds of fresh parsley to make 1 pound of dried, yet dried parsley has only *half* the taste and minerals of fresh parsley.

Boost the Benefits

- Select healthy, fresh-looking bunches with bright green, crisp leaves.

- Keep parsley fresh by moistening a paper towel and wrapping it around the parsley bunch. Place in a plastic bag and store it in the refrigerator for up to 1 week.
- You can freshen slightly wilted leaves by standing the stems in cold water. However, this causes some loss of vitamin C.
- Like many herbs, fresh parsley can be frozen. Wash the parsley and pat it dry. After chopping it, put the parsley in a plastic bag and toss it in the freezer. When you're ready to cook it, just take out what you need. It will thaw almost immediately.
- Remember that cooking parsley for a long time takes away from its flavor and nutrient value, so add it toward the end of cooking.
- To intensify the flavor of *any* dried herb, sprinkle it over fresh parsley leaves before you chop them.

Be a Fat Flush Cook

- To reap the benefits of parsley, use it fresh by tossing a handful into your salad or sprinkling minced leaves over cooked foods.
- Mix some freshly minced parsley and garlic into flaxseed oil for a savory, yet simple, topping for steamed vegetables.
- Parsley enriches the flavor of any broth. Stir some parsley leaves—and stems—into homemade or canned broth.
- If you add too much garlic to a broth or soup, you can remove some by inserting parsley leaves into a tea infuser and placing the infuser in the broth. The parsley attracts the garlic.

It's Been Said . . .

You might want to try drying your own parsley. I spread freshly gathered parsley on a piece of parchment paper and place in a 200 degree oven with the door cracked open. As soon as the parsley is dry, I crush it and put it in a bottle with a cork stopper. The parsley stays green and flavorful this way.

SANDY S., MASSACHUSETTS

CHAPTER

6 Surprising Fat Flushing Foods

To eat is a necessity, but to eat intelligently is an art.

LA ROCHEFOUCAULD

In this chapter, you'll find foods that have earned a place on your Fat Flushing dinner plate. Some of my selections may surprise you, because they are items often omitted from the typical dieter's grocery list. However, each of these foods provides concentrated nutrition—giving you the best Fat Flushing bang for your buck.

For example, I recommend whole-fat or low-fat yogurt, rather than the fat-free varieties that are so often loaded with extra carbs and artificial sweeteners. Along with those all-important active bacterial cultures, yogurt provides calcium, which is emerging as one the latest weight loss tools. You'll also see that I've included bread (made with spelt) and potatoes (only sweet, please) as two of our Fat Flushing superfoods.

You have the power to reach your weight loss goals by eating the right kinds of Fat Flushing fats, proteins, and carbohydrates. The key to achieving a fit, toned body is to start from the inside out by cleansing the liver, revving up the metabolism, and evening out blood-sugar levels. Only then will your body be primed for optimal fat burning and weight loss. The following five foods make important contributions to your development as a lean, mean fat-burning machine.

ALMONDS

Fat Flush Factors

Cholesterol Zapper

Energizer

Blood-Sugar Stabilizer

What blooms like a peach and looks like a peach, but is harvested for its seed rather than its fruit? You guessed it—it's the almond. These oval, off-white nuts grow on trees and are technically the seeds of almond fruits. One of the earliest cultivated foods, the almond is the most nutritionally well-balanced nut. It is high in protein, contains healthy fats, and offers ample amounts of vitamin E, calcium, fiber, folate, iron, potassium, zinc, and magnesium. But there's more. Almonds are an excellent source of biotin, a B vitamin involved in the metabolism of both sugar and fat. By eating almonds, you can boost your energy, improve the health of your skin and hair, and maximize your nervous system function.

Studies have shown that people who eat almonds on a regular basis enjoy a lower risk of heart disease, have healthy blood-sugar levels, and have a good chance of shedding those excess pounds. A recent study, published by the American Heart Association, detailed the effect that almonds can have on cholesterol levels. Dieters who ate two handfuls of almonds per day saw a drop in LDL cholesterol levels of over 9 percent, compared with dieters who substituted a low-fat, whole wheat muffin for the almonds.[1] Many researchers agree that crunching on an ounce of almonds per day will reduce your risk of heart disease by 30 percent.

Because almonds contain fiber, protein, and fat, they satisfy both your appetite and the desire for something crunchy. Snacking on a small handful of almonds can help you feel fuller, longer. A recent study followed 65 overweight people, three-fourths of whom were type 2 diabetics. The group of dieters who ate 3 ounces of almonds every day dropped 18 percent of their weight in 24 weeks. The dieters who ate the same healthy menu, without the almonds, averaged only an 11 percent loss. In addition to the faster weight loss, the almond eaters saw improvement in their blood pressure readings and were able to lower their use of diabetes medications.[2] It's unmistakable.

Almonds are a high-fat food that is great for your health and your waistline.

Recommended Usage: Up to 1 ounce of almonds per day.

Just the Facts

- How long have almonds been around? Botanists believe they are a *prehistoric* hybrid of unknown origins.
- California produces 80 percent of the world's supply of almonds.
- It takes 1000 pounds of almonds to make 1 pint of almond oil.
- If you cut down an almond tree, shoots grow up from the stump and become a tree again in just a few years.
- One-fourth cup of almonds contains more protein than an egg.

Boost the Benefits

- Since almonds have a high fat content, they must be stored properly to protect them from becoming rancid. *Unshelled* almonds have the longest shelf life. When buying these, avoid shells that are split, moldy, or stained.
- Because they are not exposed to heat, air, and humidity, shelled almonds that come in a sealed container will last longer than those sold in bulk bins. When you're buying almonds from bulk bins, look for nuts with a uniform color. Avoid almonds that are limp, shriveled, or have a sharp or bitter odor. Store almonds in sealed plastic bags or glass jars. If well sealed, you can refrigerate almonds for several months, or pop them in the freezer for up to 1 year.
- If you combine almonds with foods rich in vitamin C, you'll improve your body's ability to absorb iron.
- Give your bones a boost. Eating approximately 20 almonds provides you with as much calcium as 1/4 cup of milk.

Just for Fun!

A favorite snack among Japanese teenagers is a mixture of dried sardines and slivered almonds.

Be a Fat Flush Cook

- To toast your own almonds, spread them in a shallow pan and heat them in a 170 degree oven for 20 minutes. This preserves the healthy oils in the nuts.

- Sprinkle some chopped almonds over a salad or steamed vegetables.
- Skip that high-carb granola and mix some chopped almonds into your yogurt instead.
- Add crunch to your stir-fry with a handful of sliced almonds.
- A spoonful of natural almond butter added to your morning smoothie gives it extra flavor and protein.

THINK TWICE!

- *Nuts can cause hives, headaches, and other allergic reactions. People who are allergic to aspirin may react to the natural salicylates found in almonds.*
- *The commercial roasting process for nuts is a form of deep-frying, usually in saturated fat such as coconut or palm kernel oil. If you buy roasted almonds, select ones that have been "dry roasted." Check the label to be sure that no additional ingredients such as sugar, corn syrup, or preservatives have been added.*

It's Been Said . . .

I'm always looking for a healthy snack that I can pack in my purse. My latest favorite is slivered almonds and apple slices.

Susan T., Iowa

OLIVE OIL

Fat Flush Factors

Cholesterol Zapper

Detoxifier

Blood-Sugar Stabilizer

Since ancient times, the olive tree has served as a symbol of peace and has supplied people with food, fuel, and medicine. While olive oil has been consumed since 3000 B.C., it enjoyed little popularity in the United States until the 1970s. During that decade, researchers began to boast about the health benefits of olive oil, causing supermarkets to carry a sampling of olive oils from various countries.

Today, on grocery shelves, you can find a number of grades of olive oil—ranging from "premium extra-virgin" to "light." Premium extra-virgin olive oil is produced by pressing perfectly ripe olives within 24 hours of their being harvested. It contains the highest density of powerful antioxidants called *polyphenols,* known for attacking free radicals before they can do their cholesterol-raising damage.

Extra-virgin olive oil is made from the first pressing of olives, while virgin olive oil comes from olives that are slightly riper. Pure olive oil is a commercial grade blend of olive pulp, skins, and pits. Light olive oil results from the final pressing of a batch of olives and carries little of the true aroma and flavor of olive oil.

Although olive oil is a fat, it still ranks as a Fat Flushing food. It deserves this status because of its monounsaturated fat, which decreases LDL cholesterol and the risk of heart disease. In addition, the natural antioxidants in olive oil help lower cholesterol levels, maintain a healthy blood pressure and guard against the toxins that can cause breast cancer.

Because of its low acidity level, especially in the higher grades of oil, olive oil is easier to digest compared to most other fats. The high vitamin E content of olives may even help reduce the frequency and/or intensity of hot flashes in women going through menopause. And, by consuming small amounts of this good fat, you'll help satisfy your appetite and keep your blood sugar on an even keel.

Recommended Usage: Up to 1 tablespoon per day.

Just the Facts

- In ancient Greece, olive oil was so highly valued that only virgin boys were allowed to pick olives, one by one.
- Spain is the world's biggest supplier of olive oil. Some of its olive trees are over 1000 years old.
- Olive oil is always of the best quality in the year it is produced, unlike wine, which may require several years to reach its peak.
- The cost of extra-virgin olive oil ranges from $5 to $100 per quart, depending on the type of olive used, where it was cultivated, and how it was processed.

Boost the Benefits

- Air, heat, and light cause olive oil to turn rancid, so store it in a cool, dark place in a container with a tight cap. If you refrigerate it, the oil may thicken and darken, but it will return to its original, liquid state when it is warmed to room temperature. However, refrigeration may alter the flavor of extra-virgin oil, so treat it delicately.
- Once you've opened a bottle of olive oil, it begins to oxidize and is best when used within a couple of months. However, if it is stored properly, olive oil can be kept longer than any other edible oil without going rancid.
- Your best bet is to store olive oil in a glass, glazed clay, or stainless steel container. Copper or iron containers cause a chemical reaction, which damages the oil and may produce toxins. Avoid storing olive oil in plastic containers because, over time, the oil can absorb some of the compounds used in the plastic.
- Because of the higher acidity level, lower grades of olive oil have a shorter shelf life than top quality extra-virgin oil.

Be a Fat Flush Cook

- Olive oil is perfect for meat, fish, or poultry marinades. Brushing olive oil onto meats prior to broiling, grilling, or roasting will help brown the meat and seal in the juices.
- Instead of serving butter with bread, pour a bit of olive oil onto a small plate for dipping.
- Sprinkle olive oil on cooked vegetables for a satisfying flavor.
- Substituting light olive oil for butter makes for moist and tender baked goods, without risk of a heavy olive flavor. For most recipes, use 3/4 cup oil for every cup of butter.

- Tossing vegetables in olive oil before cooking seals in moisture, adds flavor, and promotes browning.
- For sautéing or baking, use light olive oil, but when mixing a salad dressing, extra-virgin olive oil is worth every penny.

Fat Flushing Fun

If you want to taste test olive oil like the experts, follow these simple steps:

1. Pour 1 tablespoon of olive oil in a small glass. Rotate the glass delicately until the oil has adhered to the entire inside surface of the glass. Warm the glass in your hands until it is close to body temperature.
2. Lift the glass to your nose and sniff rapidly and deeply three times. Try to analyze the aroma.
3. Take a small sip, but don't swallow! Roll the olive oil around in your mouth for a few seconds, then spit it out. A low-quality oil will leave an aftertaste, while high-quality extra-virgin olive oil will leave your mouth clean, with just a hint of pepper.
4. If you are sampling more than one oil, drink lots of water and eat a small piece of bread between samples.

THINK TWICE!

- *Some flavored olive oils have additives that require refrigeration in order to preserve them, so please read the label carefully. If you make your own flavored olive oils, use them immediately because some flavoring agents promote the growth of bacteria.*
- *If you purchase unfiltered olive oil, it should be consumed within a year of production. Keep in mind that it takes some time for olive oil to reach store shelves, so 6 months may have passed by the time you buy it.*
- *Some people experience a slight laxative effect from olive oil, so add it gradually to your daily diet.*

It's Been Said . . .

While on a Fat Flush Caribbean Cruise with Ann Louise, she told us how great olive oil is for the skin. She rubs olive oil on her elbows and into her cuticles. Give it a try—it really works!

LINDA L., DURHAM, NC

SPELT

Fat Flush Factors

Cholesterol Zapper

Blood-Sugar Stabilizer

In my private practice, I have evaluated thousands of clients, and the vast majority of them have been sensitive to wheat. One reason for this is that, over the decades, modern wheat has been bred to give extra volume to baked goods by having its gluten content increased. This change in wheat production has caused Americans to take a look at alternative grains, including spelt. An ancient grain, spelt enjoys worldwide popularity and is, in many ways, the ideal grain. The spelt kernel is surrounded by a tough outer husk that keeps it fresh, protects it from pollutants, and allows it to be grown without pesticides.

Unlike wheat, spelt has retained many of its original traits and offers a nutty flavor and a wealth of nutrients. Spelt is naturally high in fiber and beats wheat when it comes to protein, the B vitamins, and energy-producing complex carbohydrates. Spelt is the only grain containing *mucopolysaccharides*, a compound that stimulates the immune system.

Regular consumption of niacin and riboflavin-rich spelt helps reduces the risk for heart disease by 25 percent and stroke by 35 percent. Its high fiber content works to lower cholesterol levels and regulate both blood-sugar and insulin levels. Spelt also provides an ample amount of zinc, which assists with blood-sugar control and serves as a "body cleansing" antioxidant. Best of all, even though it contains a small amount of gluten, spelt seems to be tolerated by *most* wheat-sensitive people.

Recommended Usage: One or two slices of spelt bread per day.

Just the Facts

- The total protein content of spelt is 10 to 25 percent higher than that of commercial wheat.
- Removing that tough outer husk is an expensive process, which explains why spelt costs more than wheat.

- Because spelt has a high water solubility, its nutrients are easily absorbed by the body.
- By eating just a couple of slices of spelt bread, you'll meet nearly 20 percent of your daily fiber requirement.

Boost the Benefits

- Store spelt in a cool, dry area in a sealed glass or plastic container—to keep it away from air, moisture, and sunlight.
- Check your local health-food store for spelt products, including flour, assorted pastas, cereals, and breads. You can store these delicious breads in the freezer; just remove slices as you need them.
- You may find spelt grains and flours available for sale from bulk containers. If so, make sure that the bins containing the spelt are covered and that there is no evidence of moisture.
- You may want to look for spelt "berries," which are the hulled whole grains.

Be a Fat Flush Cook

- For a robust treat, try using spelt bread for your next sandwich.
- Spelt flour can be substituted for wheat flour in most baked goods, giving them a light, slightly sweet, and nutty flavor.
- Spelt berries may be cooked and served as you would rice or potatoes. Before cooking, rinse them thoroughly under running water to remove any dirt or debris. After rinsing, soak the berries in water for 8 hours. Drain, rinse, and then add three parts water to each part spelt. Bring to a boil, then reduce the heat, and simmer for about 1 hour.
- Add spelt flakes to tomato-based soups, or cook the whole grain with olive oil, chopped fresh rosemary, and crushed garlic. Then serve hot.

THINK TWICE!

If you have a full-fledged gluten intolerance or have been diagnosed with celiac disease, you may not be able to eat spelt products.

It's Been Said . . .

One of my favorite Fat Flush breakfasts is French toast made with spelt bread. I top it with fresh or frozen blueberries which have been heated and mashed. It's so good, it seems impossible that I can eat it and still lose weight, but I can!

DENISE R., OREGON

Spelt is the best of grains. It is rich and nourishing and milder than other grain. It produces a strong body and healthy blood to those who eat it and it makes the spirit of man light and cheerful.

SAINT HILDEGARD, THIRTEENTH CENTURY

SWEET POTATOES

Fat Flush Factors

Cholesterol Zapper

Blood-Sugar Stabilizer

It's hard to believe that a food with both "sweet" and "potato" in its name is a great food for dieters. Yet, it's true. Sweet potatoes are among the most nutritious foods in the vegetable kingdom. And, as scientists have discovered, they are also one of the oldest known vegetables, having been consumed 10,000 years ago by prehistoric people.

In the early 1900s, Americans were most familiar with the pale-fleshed sweet potato. When a new orange-colored variety was introduced, it was frequently called a "yam" to avoid confusion between the two types of sweet potatoes. However, a true yam is a large African root vegetable that can grow to be 100 pounds and is rarely found in the United States.

Despite its name, the sweet potato bears no relation to the common potato and can be eaten by people who normally steer clear of potatoes. Sweet potatoes are packed with calcium, potassium, and vitamins A, C, and E. They also provide fiber, iron, thiamine, and manganese. As an antioxidant-rich food, the sweet potato helps the body eliminate free radicals, chemicals that damage cells and promote heart disease and cancer.

Recently, sweet potatoes gained the well-deserved title of "antidiabetic food" because of their power to stabilize blood-sugar levels and lower insulin resistance. So the next time your sweet tooth rears its ugly head, skip the cakes and cookies and enjoy a delicious and satisfying sweet potato.

Recommended Usage: Two to three 1/2 cup servings per week.

Just the Facts

- Sweet potatoes contain an enzyme that contributes to its sugary flavor. This sweetness continues to increase during storage and as the potatoes are cooked.
- Despite their sweetness, sweet potatoes are considerably lower on the glycemic index than white potatoes. A baked sweet potato is 77 on the index, while a baked white potato is 121.

- Out of 400 varieties of sweet potatoes, two are most common: the pale yellow kind with dry flesh and those that are dark orange with a moist flesh. Generally, dark orange sweet potatoes are plumper and more flavorful.
- During the Civil War, coffee was scarce, so people dried sweet potatoes and ground them as a substitute for coffee.
- While sweet potatoes can be found year-round, they are in season during November and December.

Boost the Benefits

- When you're buying sweet potatoes, select potatoes that are heavy and firm with smooth, bright skin, and no cracks or bruises. Avoid potatoes on display in a refrigerated produce section because the cold can be damaging.
- Keep in mind that even if you cut away a spot of decay, it may have already given the whole potato an unpleasant flavor.
- Store sweet potatoes in a cool, dark, and well-ventilated place. Temperatures above 60 degrees cause them to sprout or ferment, while air cooler than 50 degrees triggers an unpleasant change in flavor. Keep the potatoes loose, not in a plastic bag, and they should remain fresh for at least 10 days.
- Before storing sweet potatoes, you may brush off excess dirt, but, to prevent spoilage, do not wash them until you are ready to cook them.
- Cook sweet potatoes *whole* whenever possible since most of the nutrients are next to the skin. However, because dyes and wax are sometimes used on the skin, do not eat it unless the potato has been grown organically.

Be a Fat Flush Cook

- Yellow and orange sweet potatoes may be used interchangeably in recipes; however, avoid mixing the two types as their cooking times vary.
- Purée cooked sweet potatoes with a bit of natural applesauce and cinnamon. Top with ground flaxseed.
- Cut a sweet potato into thin slices and bake to make crunchy sweet potato chips.
- Sweet potatoes can be boiled, grilled, baked, and roasted. So, don't be afraid to experiment with this versatile vegetable.
- You can freeze cooked sweet potatoes. Simply add a little lemon juice to prevent darkening and pack them into freezer containers.

THINK TWICE!

- *While canned sweet potatoes are available, they usually come in heavy syrup and are substantially lower in beta-carotene, vitamin C, and B vitamins than fresh ones.*
- *Because pesticide residues are commonly found on sweet potatoes, it's best to look for organically grown ones, whenever possible.*
- *Sweet potatoes are among the few foods that contain oxalates, which, if concentrated in the body, can crystallize and cause health problems. If you have a history of kidney or gallbladder trouble, you may want to avoid eating sweet potatoes.*
- *Oxalates may also prevent the body from absorbing calcium. If you take calcium supplements, allow 2 to 3 hours between taking your supplement and eating a sweet potato.*

It's Been Said . . .

I'm always looking for new things to pack for lunch. My latest favorite is a sweet potato, baked the night before and packed cold in my lunch bag. Yum! It's almost like having dessert.

JENNIFER B., FLORIDA

YOGURT

Fat Flush Factors

Thermogenic

Detoxifier

Energizer

Yogurt is one dairy product that I can recommend wholeheartedly. Made by adding bacterial cultures to milk, yogurt has a refreshingly tart flavor and a unique creamy texture. Because it contains beneficial bacteria, yogurt increases resistance to immune-related diseases and may help you live longer. One recent 5-year study tracked a population of 162 very elderly people and found that those who ate yogurt more than three times per week were 38 percent more likely to survive the term of the study than those who ate yogurt less than once a week.[3]

Yogurt provides ample amounts of a number of important nutrients. If you consume yogurt regularly, you'll be strengthening your bones with calcium and phosphorous, fortifying body tissues with protein, and energizing your metabolism with riboflavin and niacin. But it is the bacterial cultures—known as probiotics—that make yogurt a Fat Flushing superfood.

From minimizing bad breath to preventing yeast infections, probiotics work their magic throughout the body. They contribute to intestinal health, and, because they are resistant to stomach acid, continue their beneficial activities as they travel through the entire digestive tract. Johns Hopkins researchers found that yogurt helps reduce fatty liver disease, a common condition that is on the rise among overweight people.[4] And eating yogurt with live cultures revs up your body's ability to burn fat. A recent study at the University of Tennessee found that people who incorporated yogurt into their diet plan lost 22 percent more weight and 61 percent more body fat than people who simply reduced their caloric intake.[5] This may stem from the fact that yogurt is high in calcium, which is essential for releasing the hormones that break down fat. So how about adding a little "culture" to your life by enjoying some delicious, Fat Flushing yogurt?

Recommended Usage: Up to 1 cup of whole-fat or low-fat yogurt per day.

Just the Facts

- Americans eat over 300,000 tons of yogurt each year.
- For most people, eating 1 cup of yogurt a week is enough to keep their intestines colonized with good bacteria.
- Because of the lactase it contains, yogurt is digested three times faster than milk. This makes it well tolerated by people who are lactose-intolerant.

Boost the Benefits

- When you're shopping for yogurt, look for products that are made from organic milk and spell out which live active cultures it contains. The best quality products have the following five live bacteria: S. thermophilus, L. bulgaricus, L. acidophilus, L. casei, and L. reuteri.
- Avoid yogurts that contain artificial colors, flavorings, or sweeteners. This includes fruit-filled yogurt, which often contains excess sugar.
- Remember to check the expiration date on yogurt containers to make sure they are fresh.
- Store yogurt in the refrigerator in its original container. If *unopened*, yogurt stays fresh for about 1 week past the expiration date.

Be a Fat Flush Cook

- Yogurt can become thin and runny if it is mixed or heated too much. For best results, be careful not to stir it excessively or overheat it.
- Use plain yogurt when you're making dips for fruits and vegetables; sauces for meat, fish, and poultry; and dessert toppings.
- For a delicious dip, add chopped cucumber and fresh dill to plain yogurt.
- Give your morning smoothie a calcium boost by adding a dollop of plain yogurt.
- Have yogurt as a snack, dessert, or light meal. Try a healthy yogurt shake or use plain yogurt in place of sour cream.

THINK TWICE!

Even if you have a general intolerance for dairy products, you may be able to eat yogurt because the process of making yogurt transforms the lactose in milk into lactic acid. In studies, yogurt with active lactic acid bacteria improved lactose absorption in lactose-intolerant people. If you want to test your response to yogurt, be sure you purchase plain yogurt that contains live active cultures.

It's Been Said . . .

One of my favorite desserts is both elegant and easy. I alternate layers of yogurt and fresh berries in a large wine glass or snifter. I sprinkle ground flaxseeds on top for a bit of crunch. I've even served it at dinner parties and people love it!

PEGGY K., GEORGIA

CHAPTER

7 Fat Flushing Supplements

It is better to prepare and prevent than to repair and repent.

ANONYMOUS

Leaves, roots, flowers, bark, stems, and seeds. These are the humble sources of the Fat Flushing supplements discussed in this chapter. Giving the body a boost with natural herbs and plants is not new. The medicinal benefits of plants have been known for centuries and span all cultures. Herbs have been used throughout history as a means of enhancing health, curing illness, or preventing disease. In fact, many modern drugs are derived from the powerful active ingredients in plants.

In today's world, because of soil conditions and food production methods, we can't always get all the nutrients we need from foods—no matter how healthy our diet. I believe that certain supplements are crucial to successful weight loss and ongoing weight control. From essential and critical fatty acids to liver cleansing herbs, the following Fat Flushing supplements are your "support system," extra weapons in your arsenal against aging and weight gain.

Every year, sales of herbal supplements amount to hundreds of millions of dollars in the United States alone. And, health-food stores carry a bewildering number of items. How can you know which supplements to buy? With the supplement industry so loosely regulated, it is crucial to purchase only those products that you know to be of superior quality. Otherwise, you may not be getting what is indicated on the label—or you may be getting more, in the way of sugar, additives, fillers, and preservatives.

Many of the herbal supplements available today target specific problems, such as arthritis pain, muscle spasms, or a weak immune system. The focus of the Fat Flushing supplements is, of course, to gently support the liver while promoting fat burning and weight loss—without the use of harmful substances like ephedra or guarana. In addition, these Fat Flushing supplements all offer additional benefits that help us in our quest to be healthy and beautiful—now and in the years to come.

CHOLINE

Fat Flush Factors

Detoxifier

Cholesterol Zapper

Energizer

Before 1998, scientists believed that the human body made adequate amounts of choline. However, after additional research, the National Academy of Sciences classified choline as an essential nutrient—and acknowledged that we can't always produce the required amount. Unfortunately, coming up short on choline can lead to hypertension, arteriosclerosis, cirrhosis, and fatty deposits in the liver.

Choline is vital to controlling fat and cholesterol buildup in the body; regulating the kidneys, liver, and gallbladder; and banishing fatigue. Recent studies have concluded that choline helps the body burn fat while simultaneously lowering cholesterol. As an added bonus, choline helps form *phosphatidylcholine*, which is needed for proper mental functioning. Providing your body with adequate choline while you are young can help diminish memory deficits as you age. Choline can nourish your brain *and* your liver while it helps you lose weight. That's quite a deal.

Recommended Usage: Based on current research, a reasonable amount of choline supplementation is 250 to 1000 milligrams daily. I suggest 300 to 350 milligrams per day.

Just the Facts

- Choline is an essential nutrient sometimes referred to as vitamin B^4.
- Just a few weeks on a choline-deficient diet has been shown to cause abnormal liver function.
- The main dietary source of choline is lecithin, which is found in foods such as eggs, fish, and nuts.

Boost the Benefits

- You may want to take choline supplements early in the day because some people find that choline interferes with their sleep if taken in the evening.
- Taking choline right before a meal is fine, although it works equally well when taken with food.

CHROMIUM

Fat Flush Factors

Energizer

Blood-Sugar Stabilizer

Cholesterol Zapper

Since the 1960s, researchers have known that chromium plays a vital role in the metabolism of glucose and is needed for proper insulin function and energy production. If we don't get enough chromium, we suffer from impaired insulin activity known as "insulin resistance." As the body becomes insulin resistant, more glucose remains in the blood stream and ends up being stored as fat, rather than moving into the cells to be burned for energy. Chromium helps stabilize blood-sugar levels and is also crucial to the synthesis of cholesterol, fats, and proteins. Since overweight people are often insulin resistant, chromium is a natural choice for promoting a healthy metabolism, reducing body fat, and preserving lean muscle.

In fact, chromium is a dieter's dream supplement. It serves to suppress the appetite and reduce cravings. Additionally, it has been shown to build muscle and trim fat at the same time. A recent study, published in *Current Therapeutic Research,* reported on a group of overweight volunteers who were given 400 mcg of chromium for 72 days. Even though they followed no particular diet or exercise regime, they lost an average of over 4 pounds of fat while gaining 1.4 pounds of lean muscle.[1]

While chromium is found in tiny amounts in many foods, it is difficult to consume enough to meet our needs—especially as we get older. Lifestyle has an impact, as both strenuous exercise and a diet high in sugar cause the body to use chromium more rapidly. To make matters worse, American soil has become chromium-deficient. How can you tell if you are lacking in this essential mineral? Some of the symptoms include anxiety, coronary blood vessel disease, depression, diabetes, high cholesterol, hyperinsulinism, hypoglycemia, hyperactivity, and obesity.

Recommended Usage: The Reference Daily Intake (RDI) for chromium is 120 mcg, but clinical research suggests that 200–400 mcg are needed for optimal health benefits.

Just the Facts

- The older we get, the less chromium our bodies are able to store.
- When the body is lacking chromium, it takes *twice* as long for insulin to remove glucose from the blood.

Boost the Benefits

- Chromium works best if taken *before* meals.
- Get all the chromium you need by taking the Fat Flush Weight Loss Formula.

THINK TWICE!

- *Don't exceed a daily chromium dose of 1200 mcg because too much chromium may result in liver and kidney problems.*
- *Pregnant or breast-feeding women should avoid chromium supplements.*

It's Been Said . . .

I've lost 50 pounds and 30 inches with the help of the Fat Flush Weight Loss Formula, which includes chromium and other fat-burning supplements. The weight loss formula helped me feel full quickly so I never left the table still hungry!

Chris P., Virginia

CLA

Fat Flush Factors

Energizer

Blood-Sugar Stabilizer

A powerful tool for dieters, CLA, or *conjugated linoleic acid*, offers profound fat loss and healing benefits. This necessary fatty acid helps reduce body fat while retaining lean muscle mass and is an important building block for cellular growth. Before the 1970s, Americans didn't need to worry about supplementing their diets with CLA since dairy products and meats contained ample amounts naturally. But, today, because livestock is no longer grass fed, our intake of CLA has dropped by 80 percent. People who have shied away from eating meat and dairy products because of their fat content have further compounded this deficiency. Fortunately, researchers discovered a way to create CLA from the linoleic acid found in sunflower and safflower oils, and CLA is now available in a convenient capsule form.

Why is CLA such a boon to waist watchers? Study after study has shown its effectiveness in reducing body fat. The *Journal of Nutrition* published the results of the first human clinical trial using CLA, which showed a dramatic 20 percent decrease in body fat, with an average loss of 7 pounds of fat in the group taking CLA. These results were achieved without a single change in dietary habits, establishing CLA supplementation as a simple, effortless weight loss tool.[2] Another recent clinical trial, conducted at the University of Wisconsin, assessed the effects of CLA on the body composition of 80 obese men and women. All the participants dieted for several months, lost weight, and then returned to their old eating habits. While the group taking CLA did regain some weight, they put the pounds back on in a ratio of half fat to half lean muscle, compared with 75 percent fat to 25 percent muscle for the control group.[3] This evidence suggests that CLA increases lean muscle mass and results in a stronger, healthier body.

The benefits of CLA do not stop at weight loss. Over the past two decades, researchers have found that CLA also modulates the immune response, protects against heart disease, and inhibits the growth of various cancers. It may also prevent and control adult onset diabetes, a disease running rampant in our overweight country. And, because it helps prevent bone loss, CLA may also be a potent agent for preventing osteoporosis and osteoarthritis. The message is clear: Along with a balanced diet and a daily exercise program, CLA can help you fight disease and pare off the pounds.

Recommended Usage: Three to six grams daily, taken before or with meals.

Just the Facts

- CLA was first discovered in 1987 by researchers at the University of Wisconsin in Madison.
- CLA permeates muscles cells, where it has been shown to increase muscle mass by as much as 5 percent.
- You'd need to eat 6 pounds of steak or 50 slices of Colby cheese to receive the same amount of conjugated linoleic acid found in most CLA dietary supplement products.

Boost the Benefits

- Occasionally, people find that if they take CLA close to bedtime they have trouble falling asleep. I recommend that you experiment and see how your body reacts. Most people can take CLA after a late dinner and have no problems sleeping.
- It's best to avoid taking CLA with fiber supplements or high-fiber meals because the fiber may absorb some of the CLA. For best results, take CLA an hour or so after a high-fiber meal or fiber supplements.
- For weight management, most people report noticeable results after taking CLA for about 6 weeks.

GLA

Fat Flush Factors

Energizer

Thermogenic

Since the 1980s, many studies have focused on the power of GLA, or *gamma linolenic acid*, to serve as a natural aid to weight loss. Found naturally in seed oils, such as borage, evening primrose, and black currant seed oils, GLA is an essential fatty acid, which triggers fat burning instead of fat storage by boosting the metabolism in two ways: First, it fuels the burning of brown adipose tissue, a type of fat commonly dormant in overweight people. Second, it stimulates a metabolic process commonly referred to as the "sodium pump," helping to use up nearly half of the body's calories.

In a healthy body, GLA can be synthesized from linoleic acid, which is found in certain oils, grains, and seeds. But because of a number of common dietary and lifestyle factors in today's society, most of our bodies don't make that conversion. The main metabolic roadblocks are artificial transfats, sugar, smoking, alcohol, aging, and illnesses such as diabetes. All these factors affect the body's ability to convert linoleic acid into GLA and efficiently burn fat.

Luckily, it's easy to give your body the GLA it needs to become an efficient fat-burning machine. GLA is found naturally in seed oils like borage oil (20–24 percent GLA), evening primrose oil (8–10 percent GLA), and black currant seed oil (about 15 percent GLA). Supplementing with these oils provides GLA in a usable form, so the body can bypass the conversion process and get down to the business of burning excess fat.

Like other fatty acids, GLA is thought to help to elevate levels of serotonin, a brain chemical that contributes to the feeling of fullness. This is perhaps the reason why you will feel satisfied sooner, which puts the brakes on the urge to overindulge.

The benefits of GLA extend beyond weight loss. It also controls PMS symptoms, lowers high blood pressure, wards off rheumatoid arthritis, and may help certain drug-resistant cancers. And, a steady supply of GLA helps skin retain its moisture and stay supple and smooth.

Recommended Usage: The recommended dose of GLA ranges from 300 to 2000 milligrams per day. I suggest 360 mg, taken in two daily doses of 180 mg each.

Just the Facts

- Medical studies from around the world make it clear that nearly every area of the body can benefit from GLA supplementation.
- Essential fatty acids, including GLA, were "uncovered" by scientists during the 1980s.

Boost the Benefits

- It may take 3 to 6 weeks before you feel the full effects of GLA supplementation.
- GLA is most effective when taken in two divided daily doses.
- Take GLA with food to enhance its absorption and minimize the likelihood of digestive upset.
- Like other polyunsaturated fats, evening primrose, black currant, and borage oils are easily oxidized and can spoil when exposed to heat, light, and oxygen. Even softgels, which are designed to prevent oxidation, can turn rancid. Store them in a cool, dry place away from light.
- Do not cook with GLA oils. They will break down and become ineffective if exposed to high heat.

THINK TWICE!

- *If you take prescription blood thinners, such as warfarin, check with your doctor before taking evening primrose oil. This form of GLA may impair the ability of your blood to clot.*
- *Rancid GLA products often taste or smell "funny" and are more likely to cause digestive upset.*

L-METHIONINE

Fat Flush Factors

Thermogenic

Detoxifier

Cholesterol Zapper

An essential amino acid, L-methionine teams up in your body with choline and inositol to form a powerful trio of nutrients that assists in the breakdown of fats. L-methionine helps lower cholesterol levels by increasing the liver's production of lecithin. At the same time, it prevents excess fat buildup in the liver and is an excellent detoxifier, ridding the body of heavy metals such as lead, cadmium, and mercury.

Through its supply of sulfur, L-methionine protects cells from airborne toxins, such as smog. This helps prevent disorders of the hair, skin, and nails, all the while slowing down the aging process. This little amino acid also protects the kidneys by creating ammonia-free urine. In a recent study of women with recurring urinary tract infections, L-methionine was found to prevent bacteria from adhering to the cells of the urinary tract, thereby sparing the women from yet another bladder infection.[4]

Because the body can't produce L-methionine, we have to get it from food or supplements. To ensure adequate daily amounts, I recommend supplementation.

Recommended Useage: 100 mg per day.

Just the Facts

- Small daily amounts of methionine are enough for most people to maintain good health.
- L-Methionine can be found in meat, eggs, onions, beans, lentils, and yogurt.

Boost the Benefits

- You'll benefit most from L-methionine if you take it before meals.

- L-methionine is most effective when your body has an adequate supply of magnesium. So be sure you're getting at least 400 milligrams of magnesium per day.

THINK TWICE!

Studies have shown that cancer patients should not take L-methionine because of its tendency to feed tumors.

MILK THISTLE

Fat Flush Factor

Detoxifier

Did you know that weight gain, cellulite, and abdominal bloating are just a few of the signs that the liver is overburdened? It's true. When your liver is sluggish, every organ in your body is affected, and your weight loss efforts are blocked. Some common reasons why the liver gets overloaded include environmental toxins, processed foods, overeating, and damaging factors such as alcohol, contraceptive pills, candida, and caffeine.

But, there's good news! One of the world's most thoroughly studied herbs, milk thistle, is a powerful antioxidant that has been shown to support detoxification of the liver, speed up liver function, and help regenerate new, healthy liver cells. It also changes the makeup of bile, helping to reduce the risk of gallstones.

A member of the sunflower family, milk thistle gets its strength from a complex compound called *silymarin*, which scavenges free radicals and inhibits free-radical production. Silymarin defends the liver against toxins by changing the structure of liver cells so that toxins can't get it, thereby protecting and curing the liver at the same time. So support your liver and improve your chances to lose weight with a daily dose of milk thistle.

Recommended Usage: 200 milligrams per day.

Just the Facts

- Milk thistle has been used medicinally for more than 2000 years and has been the subject of clinical trials for over 40 years.
- It is not uncommon to find milk thistle growing wild in a variety of settings, including by the side of the road. (But you should "harvest" your milk thistle in the form of a quality supplement.)

Boost the Benefits

- Although milk thistle is available as a tea, you're better off taking it in capsule or tablet form. Milk thistle is not particularly water soluble, so steeping it in a tea diminishes its liver-protective benefits.

- While milk thistle may be purchased as a "stand alone" supplement, it is absorbed better when combined with choline. You may purchase the two separately and take them at the same time, or you may find a supplement that combines the two.

THINK TWICE

Since milk thistle boosts liver and gallbladder activity, it may have a mild laxative effect in some people. This usually lasts for only 2 to 3 days.

OREGON GRAPE ROOT

Fat Flush Factors

Detoxifier

Cholesterol Zapper

Energizer

Long known as a "liver tonic," Oregon grape root is a tall shrub found in the western regions of Canada and the United States. Early American physicians learned about the medicinal benefits of grape root from the Native Americans who used it to cure a number of ailments. Now scientists know that it is the *berberine* in Oregon grape root that prevents infections by boosting the immune system and destroying bacteria. Grape root purifies the blood by activating infection fighting blood cells known as *macrophages.*

In addition, Oregon grape root stimulates the liver, gallbladder, and thyroid gland. By enhancing the flow of bile through the liver and gallbladder, grape root helps the liver filter out toxins effectively. However, the benefits of grape root don't stop there. It is also used to treat parasites, arthritis, menstrual cramps, skin diseases, and digestive problems. And because of its energizing effect on the thyroid gland, Oregon grape root fights overall fatigue, thereby helping people regain a youthful vitality.

Recommended Usage: 200 mg daily.

Just the Facts

- *Barberry* is another name for Oregon grape root.
- Oregon grape root contains anticancer compounds called *dehydropodophyllotoxin* and *podophyllotoxin.*

THINK TWICE!

- *Oregon grape root is not recommended for use during pregnancy and lactation.*
- *The effectiveness of certain medications, such as doxycycline and tetracycline, may be lessened when taken at the same time as grape root.*
- *High doses of Oregon grape root may interfere with B vitamin metabolism.*

CHAPTER

8 Fat Flushing on a Budget

The odds of going to the store for a loaf of bread and coming out with ONLY a loaf of bread are three billion to one.

ERMA BOMBECK

Ask any college student. Prepackaged, processed foods tend to be easier on the wallet than fresh produce and lean cuts of meat. Unfortunately, those inexpensive "convenience" foods provide little in the way of nutrition, are often high in carbohydrates and calories, and contain a host of unwelcome artificial ingredients.

The good news is that it is possible to pinch pennies and eat nutritious, Fat Flushing meals at the same time. I've compiled a variety of tips and practical suggestions for saving money at the supermarket while still providing your body with the Fat Flushing superfoods it deserves.

GENERAL TIPS

- Get in the habit of planning a weekly menu. This requires you to have foods on hand, causing you to make fewer trips to the grocery store. Planning also helps you make good use of leftovers, slashing both your cooking time and food costs.
- Avoid shopping for food on an empty stomach. Hungry shoppers buy more than they need.
- To keep from having to discard spoiled produce, use this book as a guide for knowing how long each food may be stored.
- Label foods with the date of purchase *before* you put them away.
- Stop buying junk food and soda. On top of being unhealthy, these items can really take a bite out of your food budget.
- Last, but not least, do what I have done for years—clean your fruits, veggies, eggs, and meats with a Clorox bath, and they'll stay fresh for much longer. In addition to avoiding toxic chemicals, you'll stop that expensive practice of throwing out overripe produce.

Food Group	Bathing Time
Leafy vegetables	15 minutes
Root, thick-skinned, or fibrous vegetable	30 minutes
Fruits	30 minutes
Poultry, fish, meat, and eggs	20 minutes

I introduced the Clorox bath back in 1988 in my first book, *Beyond Pritikin*. Based on the research of my mentor, Dr. Hazel Parcells, this simple soak not only cleanses foods, but it rejuvenates them and enhances their natural flavors.

Please note that Clorox is not the same as chlorine. In fact, the active ingredient in Clorox, sodium hypochlorite, breaks down into salt and water. The Clorox bath has been around for decades, our State Department has recommended it for military families stationed overseas. To ensure quality, use only the brand name Clorox. (Dr. Parcells was very clear that other brands were not effective.) Use 1 teaspoon of Clorox to 1 gallon of purified water. (If you can only find Clorox Ultra, cut the amount to 1/2 teaspoon to 1 gallon of water.) Place the foods to be treated into the bath for the designated length of time according to the following chart. (Please do not place ground meat in the bath, but frozen meat can be thawed in a Clorox bath, allowing about 20 minutes for up to 5 pounds of meat.) Remove the foods from the Clorox bath, place them in clear water for 10 minutes, and rinse. Dry all foods thoroughly and store.

FAT FLUSHING STAPLES

- Stock up on cranberries during the fall when they are plentiful in grocery stores. Store them in your freezer and make your own cranberry juice as needed.
- If fresh lemons are expensive in your area, it's fine to use bottled lemon juice. My favorite is the lemon (or lime) juice by Santa Cruz.
- Consider installing a "built-in" ceramic water filter under your sink. While you'll incur an initial cost, you'll pocket significant savings by drinking your own filtered water rather than expensive bottled water.

It's Been Said . . .

It's obvious that there are other Fat Flushers in my area because many times, when I'd go shopping for cranberry juice, the shelves at the store would be empty! I'd have to waste time going to other supermarkets and would often end up buying a different brand of juice that costs $2 more a bottle. Finally, I got smart. I asked my local store to order two cases of cranberry juice for me and asked for a discount. It worked! I order two cases every three months and the store gives me a 10% discount!

ELLEN H., NORTH CAROLINA

PROTEIN

- Buy "family-size" packages of meat, divide it into single servings, and freeze. You'll save money and always have some healthy protein handy.
- To save up to 50 percent on the cost of meat, learn to cut up chickens, bone meat, and grind your own hamburger.

VEGETABLES

- To add zest to grilled foods, save the loose skin on onions and garlic to toss them into the fire just before cooking meats or vegetables.
- Avoid buying produce at convenience stores because you will pay dearly for that "convenience." For example, you'll pay double the price for the "quick stop" cucumber than you would for the same vegetable at the supermarket.
- Make Fat Flush coleslaw a frequent side dish on your menu. Cabbage is cheaper and more nutritious than lettuce.
- Don't buy precut vegetables. You'll be paying more for less, nutritionally speaking.

FRUITS

- Slice fresh fruit in season and then freeze it. You'll be all set to make your morning smoothies—without buying those expensive bags of frozen fruit!
- Buy fresh berries in season and freeze them to enjoy at a later date.

It's Been Said . . .

I was in the bad habit of eating breakfast on the run—which meant buying a muffin and tall cup of coffee every day. I have saved money and my figure by making a switch. Now, I have a refreshing Fat Flushing fruit smoothie for breakfast. Sometimes, I even make it the night before, freeze it and grab it as I head out the door. By the time I get to work, my smoothie is the consistency of sorbet. Best of all, with the money I've saved, I've purchased some stylish, smaller clothes!

MINDY B., MINNESOTA

HERBS AND SPICES

- Don't waste fresh herbs. Freeze them before they go bad and you have to throw them away.
- Some spices can be purchased in bulk for a lot less money. Be sure to check for the freshness of any bulk items before parting with your money.
- Don't toss out fresh ginger peels. Freeze them for later use in soups or broth.
- Experiment with all the Fat Flushing herbs and spices. Seasonings help you economize by enhancing the taste of simple staple foods.

SURPRISING FAT FLUSHING FOODS

- Almonds are "in season" in midsummer, so stock up on fresh bulk almonds at that time, seal them, and stick them in the freezer for year round use.
- Save any leftover spelt bread and turn it into bread crumbs. Use a blender or food processor to make very fine crumbs, and then freeze them in plastic bags for later use.
- Buy plain yogurt (with live active cultures, of course), and flavor it yourself with your favorite Fat Flushing fruit.

Above all, as you prepare your grocery list, keep in mind the connection between your health and the food you eat. In this regard, a simple old saying comes to mind: "You can pay now, or you can pay later." That fast food burger off the dollar menu might seem like an inexpensive lunch, but it could cost you dearly in the long run. On the other hand, establishing eating habits that incorporate many or all of my 50 Fat Flushing foods, may help you avoid future medical expenses—and keep you slim, trim, and toned in the process.

Fat Flush Support and Resources

Here are some of the most reliable and solid resources for a variety of weight-loss–related areas ranging from Fat Flush support to recommended reading.

Support Site and Other Resources

On the Web: www.fatflush.com

I invite you to check out this Web site where you will now find a Fat Flush Store that is updated regularly with all the products that have the Fat Flush seal of approval; The Fat Flush Kit (The Dieter's Multi, GLA 90, and The Weight Loss Formula); Fat Flush Whey Protein Powder, Health From The Sun High Lignan Flaxseed Oil, Health From The Sun High Lignan Flaxseed Oil capsules, flaxseed grinders, The Woman's Oil, CLA 1000, Ultra H-3 (for depression), Y-C Cleanse (for yeast control), Super GI Cleanse, SteviaPlus (recommended sweetener), Teeccino (the herbal coffee substitute). My calendar is updated regularly on this site, so you can keep track of my media events, lectures, and radio and TV appearances.

On the Web: www.fatflush.com/forum/

And of course, you are most cordially invited to become part of our Fat Flush Forum where your nutrition and weight loss questions can be posted. This forum is supported by outstanding veteran Fat Flush Moderators who are constantly in touch with Fat Flush Fitness expert, Joanie Greggains, and me.

You are also most welcome to stop by and visit the www.ivillage.com/diet/fatflush interactive messaging board for further support, ideas, and motivation every day of the week, 365 days a year. This board is also supported by veteran Fat Flush community leaders who are in touch with me on a regular basis.

Uni Key Health Systems
P.O. Box 2287
Hayden Lake, ID 83835
800-888-4353
www.unikeyhealth.com
unikey@unikeyhealth.com

As a convenience for my many readers and clients, Uni Key Health Systems has been the official distributor of Fat Flush and related health-care products, books, and services over the years. Uni Key is the fulfillment center for The Fat Flush Store.

Joanie Greggains
P.O. Box 2708
Sausalito, CA 94966
415-332-8566
e-mail: joaniegreggains@aol.com
website: www.joaniegreggains.com

Listen to Fat Flush Fitness expert and coauthor Joanie Greggains on the radio each Saturday morning. Her show is "live" from 8–10 A.M. (Pacific time), on KGO Radio (810 AM) in Northern California, or you may listen via the Internet at www.kgo.com.

OTHER FAT FLUSH BOOKS

Here is a listing and a brief description of books that are excellent companions for your Fat Flush journey.

The Fat Flush Plan
Ann Louise Gittleman, MS, CNS
McGraw-Hill, 2002

The Fat Flush Plan is the *USA Today* and *New York Times* bestseller that melts fat from hips, waist, and thighs in just 2 weeks and reshapes your body while detoxifying your system.

The Fat Flush Cookbook
Ann Louise Gittleman, MS, CNS
McGraw-Hill, 2002

The Fat Flush Cookbook is the companion cookbook to the national bestseller, which offers more than 200 recipes for fast breakfasts, one-dish luncheons and dinners, plus snacks and scrumptious desserts using a wide variety of Fat Flushing foods, drinks, and culinary herbs and spices to cleanse and slim the body.

The Fat Flush Journal and Shopping Guide
Ann Louise Gittleman, MS, CNS
McGraw-Hill, 2003

The Fat Flush Journal and Shopping Guide is your handy, take-anywhere companion to *The Fat Flush Plan* that helps you to record your progress, weight loss, and future goals. It helps you track meals, supplements, and exercise and inspires you with daily motivational messages.

The Fat Flush Fitness Plan
Ann Louise Gittleman, MS, CNS,
and Joanie Greggains
McGraw-Hill, 2003

The Fat Flush Fitness Plan is my revolutionary program for fitness seekers, whether they are followers of the Fat Flush Plan or simply people looking for a low-impact and efficient way to exercise.

Building on the workout component of the three-phase Fat Flush Plan, fitness expert, Joanie Greggains, and I designed three distinct weight loss/maintenance sections that target the lymphatic system, which helps to flush away fat. From rebounding, walking, and weight training to specially designed yoga stretches and deep-breathing exercises, this plan will help:

- Break through workout plateaus
- Reduce tummy fat and underarm jiggles
- Ease symptoms of osteoporosis, arthritis, and diabetes
- Boost the metabolism
- Increase energy, flexibility, and strength

Used in conjunction with *The Fat Flush Plan*, this fitness plan builds calorie-burning muscle mass, speeds weight loss, and helps keep those excess pounds from returning. Throughout, readers will also find personal anecdotes from Fat Flushers, motivational tidbits, easy-to-read charts, and personal success stories.

References and Notes

General References

- Paul C. Bragg and Patricia Bragg, *Apple Cider Vinegar* (Santa Barbara, CA: Health Science, 1995).
- Ann Louise Gittleman, *Eat Fat, Lose Weight Cookbook* (Los Angeles: Keats Publishing, 2001).
- Ann Louise Gittleman, *The Fat Flush Plan* (New York: McGraw-Hill, 2002).
- Nikki Goldbeck, *The Supermarket Handbook* (New York: The New American Library, 1976).
- Ben Charles Harris, *Kitchen Medicines* (New York: Simon & Schuster, 1973).
- Lorna R. Vanderhaeghe, *Healthy Fats for Life* (Ontario: Quarry Health Books, 2003).
- Bernard Ward, *Healing Foods from the Bible* (Boca Raton, FL: American Media Mini Mags, 2001).
- Rebecca Wood, *The New Whole Foods Encyclopedia* (New York: Penguin Books, 1999).

Notes

Chapter 1

1. Amanda Buller, Arizona State University, presented at annual conference of American College of Nutrition in Orlando, FL, Oct. 6, 2001.
2. Ann Louise Gittleman, *The Fat Flush Plan* (New York: McGraw-Hill, 2002), 35.
3. John and Jan Belleme, *Culinary Treasures of Japan* (Garden City Park, NY: Avery Publishing Group Inc., 1992).
4. C. B. Pedersen, et al., "Effects of blueberry and cranberry juice consumption on the plasma antioxidant capacity of healthy female volunteers," *European Journal of Clinical Nutrition* 54 (2000): 405–408.
5. R. Goodfriend, "Reduction of bacteriuria and pyuria using cranberry juice," *Journal of the American Medical Association* 272 (August 1994): 589.
6. E. I. Weiss, et al., "Inhibiting interspecies coaggregation of plaque bacteria with cranberry juice constituent," *Journal of the American Dental Association* 129 (1998): 1719–1723.
7. O. Burger, et al., "Inhibition of Helicobacter pylori adhesion to human gastric mucus by a high-molecular-weight constituent of cranberry juice," *Critical Reviews in Food Science & Nutrition* 42 (2002): 279–284.

8. http://www.edc.gov/omh/20MHWebArchives/diabetes.spotlight.htm
9. http://www.bottledwater.org/public/2002_Releases/survey2-22.htm
10. M. Tennesen, "Drink to Your Health," *Health Magazine* 14 (June 2000): 88.

Chapter 2

1. Ann Louise Gittleman, *Eat Fat, Lose Weight* (Lincolnwood, IL: Keats Publishing, 1999), 60.
2. M. Kiatoko, et al., "Evaluating the nutritional status of beef cattle herds from four soil order regions of Florida. I. Macroelements, protein, carotene, vitamins A and E, hemoglobin and hematocrit," *Journal of Animal Science* 55 (July 1982): 28–37.
3. A. Leaf, et al., "Clinical prevention of sudden cardiac death by n-3 polyunsaturated fatty acids and mechanism of prevention of arrhythmias by n-3 fish oils," *Circulation* 107 (June 2003): 2646–2652.

Chapter 3

1. http://www.pub.umich.edu/daily/1998/oct/10-01-98/news/news19.htm
2. E. B. Rimm, et al., "Folate and vitamin B^6 from diet and supplements in relation to risk of coronary heart disease among women," *Journal of the American Medical Association* 279 (May 1998): 359–364.
3. Richard A. Anderson, et al., "elevated intakes of supplemental chromium improve glucose and insulin variables in individuals with type 2 diabetes," *Diabetes* 46 (November 1997): 1786.
4. J. W. Fahey, et al., "Sulforaphane inhibits extracellular, intracellular, and antibiotic-resistant strains of Helicobacter pylori and prevents benzopyrene-induced stomach tumors," *Proceedings of the National Academy of Sciences* 99 (May 28, 2002): 7610–7615.
5. Garnett Cheney, "Rapid Healing of Peptic Ulcers in Patients Receiving Fresh Cabbage Juice," *California Medicine* 70 (1949): 10.
6. S. Agarwal et al., "Tomato Lycopene and Low-Density Lipoprotein Oxidation: A Human Dietary Intervention Study," *Lipids* 33 (1998): 981–984.

Chapter 4

1. Le Marchand, et al., "Intake of flavonoids and lung cancer," *Journal of the National Cancer Institute* 92 (2000): 154–160.
2. D. A. Pearson, et al., "Apple juice inhibits low density lipoprotein oxidation," *Life Sciences* 64 (1999): 1913–1920.
3. P. Knekt, et al., "Flavonoid intake and coronary mortality in Finland: a cohort study," *British Medical Journal* 312 (Feb. 24, 1996): 478–481.
4. N. C. Howarth, et al., "Dietary fiber and weight regulation," *Nutrition Reviews* 59 (2001): 129–139.
5. www.coolnurse.com/aroma.htm

6. Tufts University, "Researching a blueberry/brain power connection." *Tufts University Health and Nutrition Letter* 19 (March 2001): 1.
7. www. pueblo.gsa.gov/cic_text/food/bulkfibr/bulkfibr.htm

Chapter 5

1. www.naturalhealth.net.nz/ebooksnl/nl/nhc/
2. M. Yoshioka, et al., "Effects of red pepper on appetite and energy intake," *British Journal of Nutrition* 82 (1999): 115–123.
3. http://www.sciencedaily.com/releases/1999/08/990806074926.htm
4. C. L. Broadhurst, et al., "Insulin-like biological activity of culinary and medicinal plant aqueous extracts in vitro," *The Journal of Agricultural Food Chemistry* 48 (March 2000): 849–852.
5. http://www.californialung.org/spotlight/naturaltobacco.html
6. P. J. Delaquis, et al., "Antimicrobial activity of individual and mixed fractions of dill, cilantro, coriander and eucalyptus essential oils," *International Journal of Food Microbiology* 74 (March 25, 2002): 101–109.
7. V. Chithra and S. Leelamma, "Hypolipidemic effect of coriander seeds (Coriandrum sativum): mechanism of action," *Plant Foods for Human Nutrition* 51 (1997): 167–172.
8. V. Chithra and S. Leelamma, "Coriandrum sativum changes the levels of lipid peroxides and activity of antioxidant enzymes in experimental animals," *The Indian Journal of Biochemistry and Biophysics* 36 (February, 1999): 59-61.
9. G. Singh et al., "Studies on essential oils: part 10. Antibacterial activity of volatile oils of some spices, *Phytotherapy Research* 7 (November 16, 2002): 680–682.
10. Yoshioka, "Effects," 115–123.
11. S. N. Ostad et al., "The effect of fennel essential oil on uterine contraction as a model for dysmenorrhea, pharmacology, and toxicology study, *Journal of Ethnopharmacology* 76 (August 2001): 299–304.
12. H. K. Berthold, et al., "Effect of a garlic oil preparation on serum lipoproteins and cholesterol metabolism: a randomized controlled trial," *The Journal of the American Medical Association* 279 (1998): 1900–1902.
13. B. Fuhrman, et al., "Ginger extract consumption reduces plasma cholesterol, inhibits LDL oxidation and attenuates development of atherosclerosis in atherosclerotic, apolipoprotein E-deficient mice," *The Journal of Nutrition* 130 (2000): 1124–1131.
14. E. Colquhoun, "Pungent principles of ginger (Zingiber officinale) are thermogenic in the perfused rat hindlimb," *The International Journal of Obesity* 16 (1992).

Chapter 6

1. G. E. Fraser, "Nut consumption, lipids, and risk of a coronary event," *Clinical Cardiology* 22 (July 1999): III11-5.

2. M. Wien, "Almonds vs. complex carbohydrates in a weight reduction program," *International Journal of Obesity* 27 (November 2003): 1356–1372.
3. C. Fortes, et al., "Diet and overall survival in a cohort of very elderly people," *Epidemiology* 11 (July 2000): 440–445.
4. http://www.hopkinsmedicine.org/press/2000/november/001113.htm
5. M. B. Zemel, et al., "Dairy (yogurt) augments fat loss and reduces central adiposity during energy restriction in obese subjects," *Federation of American Societies for Experimental Biology* 17 (2003): A1088.

Chapter 7

1. G. Kaats, et al., "A randomized, double-masked, placebo-controlled study of the effects of chromium picolinate supplementation on body composition: a replication and extension of a previous study," *Current Therapeutic Research* 59(1998): 379–388.
2. H. Blankson, et al., "Conjugated linoleic acid reduces body rat mass in overweight and obese human," *The Journal of Nutrition* 130:12(2000): 2943–2948.
3. M. W. Pariza, "Conjugated linoleic acid may be useful in treating diabetes by controlling body fat and weight gain," *Diabetes Technology and Therapy* 4 (2002): 335–338.
4. R. Funfstuck, E. Straube, et al. "Prevent reinfection by L-methionine in patients with recurrent urinary tract infection," *Med. Klin* 92 (1997): 574–581.

Index